Achieving Excellence:

Clinical Staffing for Today and Tomorrow

Christina K. Biesemeier, MS, RD, FADA

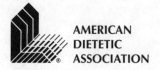

AMERICAN
DIETETIC
ASSOCIATION

Diana Faulhaber, Publisher
Jason M. Muzinic, Acquisitions Editor
Elizabeth Nishiura, Production Editor

10 9 8 7 6 5 4 3 2 1

Library of Congress Cataloging-in-Publication Data

Biesemeier, Christina.
    Achieving excellence : clinical staffing for today and tomorrow / Christina K. Biesemeier.
      p. ; cm.
    Includes bibliographical references and index.
    ISBN 0-88091-337-1
  1. Hospitals—Food service—Personnel management.   2. Health facilities—Food service—Personnel management.   3. Hospitals—Food service—Administration.   4. Health facilities—Food service—Administration.
    [DNLM: 1. Food Service, Hospital—organization & administration.   2. Personnel Staffing and Scheduling—organization & administration.   3. Efficiency, Organizational. WX 168 B589a 2004] I. Title.

    RA975.5.D5B535 2004
    362.17'6'0683—dc22

                                      2004005972

4/07   c.1

Contents

Acknowledgments

I would like to acknowledge the many dietitians and clinical nutrition managers I have met and communicated with over the years who share my vision that quality health care requires adequate dietitian and dietetic technician staffing. I commend their efforts to justify their staffing levels, often against pressure to make reductions, and to expand our profession to new levels of advanced practice.

I would like to thank the reviewers of this book, particularly Cinda Chima, MS, RD, and Ellen Pritchett, RD, CPHQ, for their valuable comments and suggestions on both the content and organization of this book, and Jason Muzinic, acquisitions editor at the American Dietetic Association, for his guidance in bringing the book to completion.

I want to thank the members of the clinical nutrition staff at the facilities where I have worked, Ochsner Foundation Hospital in New Orleans and Saint Luke's Hospital of Kansas City, and the clinical nutrition staff at Vanderbilt University Medical Center in Nashville with whom I now work. It is through their trust, support, and willingness to collect and analyze data and assume new and different roles that I have learned much of the information shared in this book.

I thank my husband, John, and children, Emily, Laura, and Steven, for their love, support, and patience in giving me the time and space to complete this book.

DEDICATION

To my husband, John, my mother and father, Mary Alice and Richard Wilburn, and my children, Emily, Laura, and Steven, with love and gratitude.

Reviewers

Cinda S. Chima, MS, RD
Director, Clinical Nutrition
Metro Health System
Cleveland, Ohio

Julie M. Finney, RD
Mercy Medical Center
Canton, Ohio

Lyn Haft, MPH, RD
Rex Health Care
Raleigh, North Carolina

Karen Hutton, RD, MA
Methodist Medical Center of Illinois
Peoria, Illinois

Bridget Klawitter, PhD, RD, FADA
All Saints Health Care
Racine, Wisconsin

Patricia Ortlieb, RD
Sodexho
St. Joseph's Wayne Hopsital
Wayne, New Jersey

Ellen Prichett, RD, CPHQ
Director, Quality and Outcomes
American Dietetic Association
Chicago, Illinois

Terri L. Thompson, RD
St. Anthony's Medical Center
St. Louis, Missouri

Introduction

Clinical nutrition staffing is extremely important for health care administrators, nutrition department directors, clinical nutrition managers, and clinical nutrition staff. Depending on whom you ask, staffing is almost always too high or too low. Rarely do you hear that staffing is just right.

One reason for these divergent viewpoints is the difference in perspectives, which range from the broad view of the administrators to the more focused view of the staff members who provide nutrition care day in and day out. However, another reason is the absence of clear definitions of desired staffing. If anything, administrators are sometimes clearer about what they want in terms of clinical nutrition staffing than are nutrition directors and managers. For administrators, appropriate staffing may be a specific level on a benchmarking report, along with the ability to provide adequate nutrition care according to the standards of the Joint Commission on Accreditation of Healthcare Organizations (JCAHO).

Nutrition directors and managers have struggled to define appropriate staffing and to support their requests for staff at levels needed to achieve positive patient outcomes. There is no validated model that is universally accepted. Often staffing is determined by budget limitations, staffing ratios that were intended to be snapshots of existing staffing rather than desired levels, and benchmarking targets. Adding to the dilemma is the variation in nutrition care procedures implemented by health care facilities in order to meet JCAHO standards.

This resource has been written to provide a comprehensive overview of clinical nutrition staffing in the inpatient and outpatient settings. It focuses on a specific subset of staff—registered dietitians and dietetic technicians—and discusses how to evaluate staffing needs and factors that affect staffing from the ground up. Even more important, it discusses how to evaluate staffing effectiveness and whether or not staffing levels are correlated with patient outcomes. It provides strategies for measuring outcomes (conducting outcomes projects and ongoing monitoring of selected clinical indicators). Content is developed around the plan-do-check-act (PDCA) performance improvement model. (Readers who would like additional information on this model or on performance measurement in general are referred to available resources such as the JCAHO publication *Tools for Performance Measurement in Health Care: A Quick Reference Guide.*

This book is divided into six chapters:

1. Assessing Staffing Needs
2. Identifying New Opportunities
3. Developing a Staffing Plan
4. Implementing a Staffing Plan and New Clinical Programs
5. Measuring and Evaluating Staffing Effectiveness
6. Clinical Nutrition Staffing: Sharing Information

Chapters 1 through 5 provide tools and forms to use in carrying out the activities that are described. Chapter 2 contains interviews with American Dietetic Association leaders and other dietitians who are practicing at an advanced level. Chapter 6 describes approaches that clinical nutrition managers have used to resolve staffing problems in their own practice settings.

The appendixes provide the tools and forms needed to plan the activities of a clinical nutrition department, evaluate requirements for the nutrition care of patients, and determine the level and type of staff to meet care requirements. Forms are also included for evaluating how well department policies and JCAHO standards for patient care are being met and for evaluating staffing effectiveness.

A theme of evidence-based practice is woven into the book. Readers are encouraged to use information from the professional literature; make data-driven decisions; and implement valid and reliable measures, procedures, and systems for nutrition care and performance measurement and management.

It is the author's vision that benchmarking systems for clinical nutrition staffing will one day include both productivity indicators and clinical effectiveness indicators. Although much work remains to be done before this vision can be achieved, if the other areas of progress made within the dietetics profession are any indicator, that day will come.

CHAPTER 1

Assessing Staffing Needs

For most managers, the process of assessing staffing needs usually starts with an evaluation of the ability of an existing staffing plan to meet existing or anticipated needs. Occasionally the process involves developing a plan for a new facility. Regardless of the point of origin, the process should be thorough, systematic, and evidence based—in other words, a planned activity that is completed within a structured model. Once initiated, the process should be repeated on a cyclical basis.

Managers can get into difficulty when the staffing assessment process is initiated in response to an urgent need, for example, a threat to reduce staff. In this situation, the goal of the process may be a quickly assembled justification of existing staff members and their positions. This approach involves two problems. First, the situation is emotionally charged, making rational decision making harder to accomplish. The second problem is that the data needed for an evidence-based approach to decision making may not exist, or they may not be collected, summarized, and organized into a format that is readily available to support logical decision making.

Managers must deliberately set aside time to plan and assess staffing needs. This activity is relatively easy to carry out when a new facility is being opened. A deadline exists, and a staffing plan must be submitted with the proposed budget. Revisions are usually made, but the need to hire and train staff in advance of the facility's opening ensures that staffing needs will be addressed.

In existing facilities, with their many demands on managers' attention, setting aside adequate time for staffing assessment is a greater challenge. An ideal time for a formal assessment is the quarter before the next annual budget is submitted. This timing allows data to be compiled and carefully reviewed. In addition, it allows time to collect additional data if needed, discuss anticipated needs with other managers, and develop proposals for new programs. To allow managers to be prepared for a formal staffing assessment, systems must be in place to support the collection of relevant data throughout the year.

TIMING A STAFFING ASSESSMENT

Although the process of assessing staffing needs involves data, numbers, and comparisons, it also requires judgment on the part of the manager. Numbers and data are vital, but so is the experience of working with people and systems. These elements will ensure that any plan developed is realistic. Managers must be connected with organizational leaders and be able to collaborate with them to meet common goals. They must be patient and realize that the seeds of future programs are sometimes planted years in advance. And they must be able to implement plans and programs and to facilitate the transitions required when assessments indicate the need for change.

ASSESSING STAFFING NEEDS: FIVE AREAS OF FOCUS

When assessing staffing needs, managers should focus their attention on five areas. These areas are described in detail later in this chapter.

1. *Facility* mission, vision, populations served, and operations
2. *Department* services and operations, with a focus on clinical nutrition services and the competencies and skill mix needed by staff
3. *Legislation* related to required patient care activities and the scope of practice of clinical nutrition staff
4. *Accreditation* standards, with a focus on identifying requirements that affect staffing, patient care, and assessment of performance
5. *Professional practice issues and guidelines* for patient care for specific patient populations

Although these five areas make up a comprehensive evaluation, each area can be evaluated separately when time permits. The goal is for managers to use an evidence-based process that is linked to their performance improvement (PI) cycle and that is practical to implement in day-to-day practice.

If a staffing plan does exist, this evaluation already may have been completed. If so, managers should update the information annually, because organizational priorities and management structures can and do change, sometimes rapidly.

Facility Overview

The first area to evaluate is the facility, which the manager should view from a broad, organizational perspective. To do so, the manager should develop an overview of the facility and its operations, as well as identify any facility characteristics that may affect staffing needs. Information can be obtained from other managers or administrators. The Healthcare Cost and Utilization Project (HCUP) databases are sources of facility data that may be available through administrators. The HCUP databases form a multistate health data system that is maintained by the Agency for Healthcare Research and Quality

(AHRQ) and used for research on the utilization of hospitals, ambulatory care centers, and outpatient facilities (1).

Each of the following areas should be considered in creating the overview. A form to use in completing the facility overview can be found in Appendix B.1.

1. Description of facility
   * Type of facility
   * Community in which the facility is located (eg, large metropolitan area, suburb of a large city, or small town)
   * Geographic area served
   * Number of beds by service (eg, medicine, surgery, obstetrics, or intensive care, and percentage of occupancy)
   * Acuity level of patients and average length of stay (ALOS) for the facility, excluding maternity patients and newborns, and by service or unit (Exclusion of maternity patients and newborns provides an ALOS that more closely depicts the ALOS of medical and surgical patients, the patients typically requiring inpatient nutrition care.)
   * Number of units and buildings
   * Relation to other hospitals (eg, part of a health care network or a free-standing facility)
   * Financial management (eg, not for profit or for profit)
   * Referral streams and relation to physicians (eg, employed physician groups, health maintenance organizations, or private practice community-based physicians)
2. Mission
   * Facility mission and values
   * Long-range goals
   * Short-term goals (eg, annual goals and organizational initiatives)
   * Budget priorities
   * Alliances
3. Patient populations
   * Ages of patients served (eg, newborns, children, adolescents, adults, and older adults)
   * Types of patients—diagnoses and conditions treated
   * Services, procedures and programs (eg, general medical and surgical care, labor and delivery, heart and kidney transplant, neonatal intensive care unit, phase II cardiac rehabilitation, subacute care, and home care)
4. Unique characteristics
   * Number and type of beds: The number and type of beds by service or unit are obtained from facility financial reports. To an extent, the size of a facility drives the need for staff; that is, more staff members are required for a large facility than a small one, other things being equal. The type of beds in a facility may affect staffing needs (eg, a large number of intensive

care beds can create a need for more staff, whereas a large number of obstetrics beds can have the opposite effect).

- Occupancy: Information on the percentage of occupancy of a facility and percentage of occupancy by service or unit within a facility is also obtained from facility financial reports. Generally, higher staffing levels are required when occupancy is higher.

- Acuity level: In general, sicker patients have greater needs, including nutrition needs, than patients who are not as sick. Facilities that provide care for patients with a high acuity level require more staff. Such facilities will have subgroups of patients whose acuity is not high. Additional staffing for the lower-acuity subgroups is not warranted based only on the overall acuity level of the facility.

- ALOS: The ALOS and acuity level are interrelated. Generally, patients with a higher acuity level have longer lengths of stay. Like the acuity level, the ALOS varies among units in a facility, based on severity of illness, complications, and co-morbidities of their patient populations.

- Number of units and buildings: Travel time and elevator access are factors in determining staffing needs.

- Relation to other hospitals: Staff members are needed both to deliver patient care and to develop systems and structures that support patient care. When a facility is part of a larger system, projects related to the delivery of patient care (eg, developing an enteral formulary) can be completed for all facilities in the system at one time, rather than by each facility. This consolidation saves considerable staff time.

- Facility mission and values: Although health care facilities provide patient care, their mission statements may be broader. For example, a mission statement may include commitment to research, teaching, and community service. These activities may increase the need for staff. At a minimum, the activities can provide a rationale for staff to be involved in them.

- Goals: Goals and initiatives can create a need for specific numbers and types of staff. Generally, short-term goals are more likely than long-range goals to drive staffing needs, because of the immediacy of the needs. At times, a facility may set a goal of achieving a quality designation (eg, a quality award or selection for inclusion on a best practice list). Although staff needs in some areas may increase as a result of this type of goal, such an increase should not be assumed. Efficiencies can be achieved that result in increased quality and decreased staffing needs.

- Budget and budget priorities: Facilities must operate within finite budgets. Because there is rarely enough money for all possible programs and initiatives, facility administrators and leaders must prioritize budget allocations. And they must make these decisions within an environment of increasing expenses of operation and decreasing revenues and reimbursement.

For example, circumstances within health care can serve as an impetus for the definition of budget priorities. An example is a nursing shortage. A facility may respond to the shortage by increasing the amount allocated for nursing salaries and sign-on bonuses. Because facility budgets are finite, increases in one area of the budget can result in downward adjustments in other areas, including nutrition services.

A nursing shortage also affects staffing in a different way. Limits on the availability of nurses force facilities to prioritize their use of the nursing staff they have. As a result, nurses are much less likely to be used for tasks that can be performed by lesser-skilled staff members (eg, tray delivery and pickup) or by other professional staff members (eg, nutrition education relating to discharge diet guidelines).

Department Overview

The second area on which to focus the staffing assessment is the nutrition department. To complete this part of the evaluation, one must develop an overview of the department and its operation, as well as identify any characteristics that may affect staffing needs. A form to use in completing the department overview can be found in Appendix B.2.

In creating the overview, consider each of the following areas:

1. Description of department
    - Position on the organizational chart and reporting relationships
    - Short- and long-term goals and how these interface with organizational goals (eg, patient satisfaction targets and revenue generation)
    - Management (eg, self-operated or contract managed, single-department director or director with multidepartment responsibilities [and, in the latter case, one site or multiple sites])
    - Relationship between foodservice and clinical nutrition services (eg, separate departments or part of the same department [and if separate, route of administrative reporting—ie, whether to the same administrator or to different administrators])
    - Levels of department management and internal reporting relationships (eg, clinical nutrition manager or self-managed clinical staff, supervisors or self-directed work teams)
    - Availability of support staff
    - Technology used (eg, automated diet office system, automated nutrition screening, on-line documentation of nutrition care, and use of hand-held devices)

- Role in training dietetic interns and other students
- Pay structure (eg, whether dietitians are exempt or non-exempt)
- Existence of a career ladder for dietitians
- Unionization

2. Scope of services and care
   - Menu system (eg, room service, select or nonselect menu cycle, and length of menu cycle)
   - Food production and delivery systems
   - Nutrition care settings (eg, inpatient coverage, outpatient clinics, and home care)
   - Nutrition care activities performed (eg, nutrition screening; nutrition assessment and reassessment; nutrition support, education, and counseling programs; and patient support groups)
   - Existence of teams for specific groups of patients (eg, nutrition support for oncology, renal, and endocrinology patients) and roles and reporting relationships of dietitians on teams
   - Indirect care activities (eg, team rounds and discharge planning meetings)
   - Nonpatient care activities (eg, PI projects and administrative duties such as menu planning and test trays)
   - Hours of operation and service, including weekend coverage and on-call services

Short- and Long-Term Goals

A strategic plan serves as the outline for department initiatives and projects. The plan often is developed through a comprehensive and structured planning process that includes the following:

- Defining or refining a mission and vision
- Analysis of factors related to department operation (eg, strengths, weaknesses, opportunities, and threats [SWOT])
- Expansion of the opportunities into program and service goals and objectives to be accomplished within a defined time (eg, the next 2 years to 3 years)

There are different approaches to strategic planning. One approach that the Joint Commission on Accreditation of Healthcare Organizations (JCAHO) has described in *Tools for Performance Measurement in Health Care* is the balanced scorecard approach (2). This approach involves setting performance goals in four broad areas: finances, customer service, internal processes, and innovation and learning. Successful performance in each area is defined, and critical measures of success are established. Measurable indicators for each area allow staff to assess progress at intervals during the time frame covered by the plan, as well as overall plan success at the end of the period. In the balanced scorecard approach, performance in all four areas is equally important, and department initiatives are expected to produce improvements in each area. A form that can be used for strategic planning using the balanced scorecard approach can be found in Appendix B.3.

Staffing is generally a component of each performance area in a strategic plan and in the goals set for each area. Examples of broad objectives that include staffing components are the opening of a new facility, the implementation of a new program (eg, a recognized diabetes self-management training program), changes in the delivery of patient care (eg, the implementation of the *ADA Medical Nutrition Therapy Evidence-Based Guides for Practice* [3]), and the implementation of an automated medical record system.

Individual department goals and plans must be established within the context of overall organizational goals and plans. For many departments, priorities include improving patient satisfaction with services, balancing expenses and revenues, and generating revenue (eg, through the use of branded foods, food and coffee kiosks, vending machines, and home meal replacement programs). Many acute care facilities are predicting decreases in patient days and accompanying reductions in reimbursement from third party payers. If these predictions are accurate, the expansion of clinical programs in the acute care setting may not be a priority or even be realistic. Existing clinical programs may even be shifted to the outpatient setting (4).

Department Management

Contract management companies may use specific systems and methods to assess staffing needs, develop staffing plans, and assess performance and productivity. These proprietary staffing models, tools, and strategies can be used in place of the models and methods described in Chapter 3.

In addition, contract management companies often provide tools and products to support patient care (eg, nutrition care manuals, educational materials, and care protocols), making it unnecessary for departments to develop their own. However, dietitians in contract-managed departments often are expected to participate on company-wide committees to review and revise existing tools and products. Although these activities are professionally rewarding, they require time.

Relationship Between Foodservice and Clinical Nutrition Services

Facilities may combine foodservice and clinical nutrition services into a single department, or they may divide the two areas, either by creating separate departments or incorporating the clinical nutrition staff into another direct patient care department. When separate, the two

---

Strategic Planning—Balanced Scorecard Approach

1. For each department initiative, set performance goals in four broad areas:
   - Finances
   - Customer service
   - Internal processes
   - Innovation and learning
2. Define critical measures of success in each of the four areas.
3. Collect performance data in each area.
4. Evaluate performance data. Performance in one area should not occur at the expense of performance in another area.
5. Use the results of the data evaluation to improve performance.

Source: Adapted from *2003 Hospital Accreditation Standards: Tools for Performance Measurement in Health Care: A Quick Reference Guide.* Oakbrook Terrace, Ill: Joint Commission Resources; 2002:246–247, with permission from Joint Commission Resources.

areas may report to the same administrator or to different administrators (eg, foodservice to a service area administrator and clinical nutrition services to a direct care administrator).

Generally, if the two areas are separate, the clinical staff has limited participation in foodservice-related activities; if the areas are united in a single department, however, clinical staff involvement in these activities tends to be greater. Such activities include planning modified menus, menu analysis, conducting meal rounds to identify changes in food preferences and to assess patient satisfaction with services, conducting test trays for compliance with quality standards, and participating on foodservice-related PI committees. Members of the clinical staff are often considered to be the eyes and ears of the department on the patient care units. As such, they provide valuable information.

Although foodservice-related activities are important to overall department function, they require time to complete, whether by clinical staff or others. Each facility must decide how to balance involving clinical staff in foodservice activities and allocating their time to direct and indirect nutrition care of patients. The staffing plan should reflect these decisions.

Levels of Department Management and Internal Reporting Relationships

Initiatives to reduce hospital and department expense budgets have resulted in the removal of one or more layers of management positions in some facilities. As a result, facilities may rely on fewer layers of managers and supervisors than they did in the past. Some departments are using self-managed teams or teams with lead staff to coordinate their work.

The extent of downsizing that has taken place has not been well reported. This problem may be due to a lack of valid and reliable tracking mechanisms and the difficulty that exists in comparing facilities. For information, managers must rely on the self-reported data from a small number of surveys, along with the anecdotal reports of other managers and clinical dietitians that are shared at professional meetings, on professional electronic mailing lists, and through informal communications.

Although potentially promoting efficiencies of time use, downsizing and the use of self-directed teams do not necessarily reduce the amount of work to be done. Staff can work harder, but there are limits to how much individuals can and will do. Generally, the duties of the downsized positions and of remaining positions are reprioritized. The result is either an elimination of low-priority duties or an extension of time lines for completion of work.

The clinical staffing plan needs to allow adequate time for clinical management duties that staff members are expected to perform as a result of downsizing (eg, self-scheduling, auditing charts, and participating on department and facility committees).

Availability of Support Staff

Another result of efforts to reduce health care costs has been a reduction in food production and support staff at some facilities. As with downsizing, data on overall reductions in staffing are limited. One survey of ADA members indicated that approximately two thirds had witnessed reductions in food production staff at their facilities as a result of cost reduction activities (5). Nearly 30% had noted a reduction in diet clerks, and approximately 20% had noted a reduction in dietetic technicians. Of interest is the fact that approximately 40% of the respondents selected "not applicable" for the question on dietetic technician reductions, suggesting that dietetic technicians were not employed at their facilities. Survey respondents were asked to compare their prereduction and postreduction duties. Many agreed or strongly agreed that after reductions were made, they were performing more administrative duties (47.6%), clerical duties (46.5%), and dietetic technician duties (42.2%).

Technology

The availability of automated systems for menu processing, nutrition care, and documentation affects staffing needs. Although health care may have been slow to automate initially, progress is being made. Implementation of systems involves a learning curve; however, once staff members are accustomed to the use of technology, efficiencies can be achieved. Applications in the inpatient clinical area include the streamlining of nutrition screening; generation of nutrition assessment documentation using data entered into automated programs via hand-held devices and desktop computers; and automatic plotting of laboratory data, growth charts, and data trends. In the outpatient setting, laboratory results can be accessed on-line. Patients with access to Web-based programs or with programs on their personal computers or hand-held devices can analyze their own food intake and e-mail the results to the dietitian in advance of their appointments. And data from similar groups of patients can be aggregated, analyzed, and compiled into reports using computer programs, making it easier to track and monitor the outcomes of medical nutrition therapy (MNT) and other types of nutrition care.

Intern and Student Training

Time for interacting with interns and students should be included in a staffing plan. The amount allocated depends on the number of staff and students involved and the nature of the precepting relationship (eg, whether an intern spends a short amount of time or an entire rotation with a dietitian and whether the rotation lasts a few weeks or an entire semester).

Some administrators and department directors question the time spent in training and express concern that training reduces time spent on patient care. Others understand that interns and students who have been trained at a facility are a pool from which vacancies can be filled, either immediately upon completion of training or in the future. In addition, positive working relationships with intern directors and instructors can lead to referrals of potential candidates for open positions.

Pay Structure

The status of dietitian positions varies among facilities; at some facilities they are exempt, and at others they are not. At facilities where the dietitians are exempt, they may be expected to work on projects and perform additional activities to support department operation. When downsizing occurs, these assignments may expand. However, as noted earlier, there are limits to the amount of additional work that can be assigned without restructuring the workload. Routine overtime for nonexempt staff is usually discouraged because of the negative impact that overtime can have on a budget, although in times of staff shortage, overtime may be used to ensure continuity in patient care.

Career Ladder

Salary is an important issue for many dietitians. Specifically, salaries do not always meet expectations based on the education and training required for the profession (6). Various strategies have been used within facilities to address the salary issue. One strategy is to establish multiple levels of dietitian positions within a department and offer additional compensation for advanced degrees and certifications. Another strategy is to create career ladders that define advanced practice roles and confer clinical privileges, such as writing orders for changes in nutrition support and tests needed to monitor nutrition support.

In the 1990s, during downsizing initiatives, the creation of multiple levels of staff and career ladders was less popular because of the vulnerability it produced for staff at higher levels in these structures. However, in the current environment, many facilities are developing structures that reward training and experience. Existing career ladder structures vary from one facility to another. Some have fewer positions at progressive steps on the ladder, making it necessary for a vacancy to occur at the next step before a qualified dietitian can move up. Other facilities allow any member of the staff who meets the specified qualifications to achieve the top step on the ladder.

Ideally, a career ladder creates a structure that combines increased requirements for training, experience, and credentials with increased responsibilities for patient care. When a career ladder is created this way, it is a tool to use in developing the staffing plan. Staff needs can be determined based on the types of patients admitted to the facility or seen for MNT in the outpatient clinics. For example, in a facility with a career ladder, coverage of intensive care units and other specialized units, such as the bone marrow transplant unit and the inpatient dialysis unit, is assigned to dietitians at a higher level on the career ladder. These dietitians are required to have advanced degrees and certifications, such as certified nutrition support dietitian (CNSD) or certified

Career Ladders

The presence of a career ladder that links successive levels on the ladder with increasing performance expectations is a win-win situation for both staff and patients.

For staff, a career ladder promotes the following:

- Development of additional knowledge, skills, and competencies.
- Use of knowledge and skills to provide patient care.
- Recognition by colleagues and the facility.

For patients, a career ladder encourages assignment of staff based on patients' needs, which promotes enhanced quality of care and improved patient safety.

specialist in renal disease (CSR). Coverage of general medicine and surgical units is assigned to dietitians at a lower level on the ladder, who are not required to have advanced degrees and certifications.

Professional issues that can surface with the use of career ladders include the limitations in practice placed on entry-level dietitians and dietitians lower on a ladder, as well as whether these limitations are consistent with the competencies established by the Commission on Accreditation for Dietetics Education (CADE). It can be argued on the one hand that the dietetics profession is a generalist one because of the broad education and training required, and that distinguishing some positions from others makes staffing more difficult. On the other hand, with the ever-expanding amount of information available, the difficulty professionals have in maintaining competence in multiple areas, and the desire of many for recognition of an advanced level of practice, specialization seems to be a worthwhile goal. In addition, facilities that link career ladder qualifications and competency assessment of staff to meeting identified patient needs for nutrition care are able to show JCAHO a strategy that demonstrates their commitment to patient safety.

The structure of the ladder has budget implications, because having more staff at higher levels on a ladder increases the amount needed for salaries. In the short term, budget predictions of the additional amount needed for salaries can be calculated using specified differences in salary from one level of the career ladder to the next (eg, 3% differences) and projections for annual increases provided by administrators or HR staff. More important, nutrition managers need to be prepared to justify the higher amounts of salaries for staff on a career ladder, because a review of salary costs in the budget can prompt administrators to request reductions in staff.

Ultimately, facility size, populations served, and care settings determine the need for advanced-level practitioners. However, what determines the likelihood of their approval, implementation, and ongoing maintenance is the ability of clinical nutrition managers and members of the clinical nutrition staff to justify the need for alternate practice and pay structures, develop workable systems, and navigate through the HR policies and procedures.

Unionization

Where unions exist, salaries are negotiated and limits on workload may be established. If workload limits are in place, staffing may be adjusted upward to comply with these limits. However, if higher salaries have been negotiated and workload limits are not in place, budget constraints may limit the number of staff employed.

Nutrition Care Settings

Hospitals have traditionally employed dietitians and dietetic technicians in relatively large numbers compared with the numbers employed in other health care settings. This situation is due in large part to the inclusion of inpatient nutrition services as a covered service in the diagnosis-dependent bundled reimbursement that facilities receive for patient care, the requirements for nutrition care established by the Centers for Medicare and Medicaid Services (CMS) as conditions for participation, and the standards for quality care established by JCAHO.

In recent years, data in the ADA membership database have indicated a downward trend in the percentages of both dietitians and dietetic technicians employed in the inpatient setting. However, absolute numbers during the most recent interval of data collection, 1997 to 1999, were slightly increased for both dietitians and dietetic technicians. Of interest is the increase in the absolute numbers of dietitians employed in clinics or ambulatory care settings and extended care facilities during the past decade. The number of clinic and ambulatory care dietitians more than doubled, representing nearly 12% of employed dietitians, and the number of dietitians employed in extended care facilities nearly doubled, representing almost 11% of employed dietitians (7).

Data from the ADA 2002 Dietetics Compensation and Benefits Survey provide support for the trends identified in the 1999 ADA membership database. These data demonstrate similar proportions of dietitians employed in the three settings (33% in hospitals, 10% in clinics or ambulatory care centers, and 10% in nursing homes) (8).

Nutrition Care Activities

Facilities are required by JCAHO and CMS to perform defined nutrition care functions to maintain accreditation and licensure. However, implementation of the standards and regulations varies from one facility to another, a factor that can have a major impact on staffing needs. (Box 1.1 summarizes factors to consider when evaluating staffing needs for nutrition care.)

Assignment of responsibility for nutrition screening is one example of variation. At some facilities, nutrition screening is incorporated into the admission assessment. Nurses or other support staff members ask nutrition screening questions during the information-gathering process prior to or on admission. When identified, indicators of nutritional risk will trigger the sending of "consult" orders to clinical nutrition staff to initiate further evaluation of the patient's nutritional status. The process may be manual, automated, or a combination of the two. If automated, the process may include the on-line comparison of selected subjective and objective data to specific, measurable criteria; automatic identification of nutritional deficits or excesses; and recommendations of consultations with clinical nutrition staff that identify the area or areas of risk.

At other facilities, nutrition staff members have responsibility for all or part of the nutrition screening process, which may be done manually or by using automated diet office systems. Nutrition screening may be assigned to dietetic technicians, when they are available. When

---

Box 1.1   Factors to Consider in Evaluating Nutrition Care

- Completion of nutrition screening
  - ➤ Staff involved
  - ➤ Adherence to procedures
- Use of technology
  - ➤ Collection and evaluation of patient data
  - ➤ Documentation of nutrition assessments and plans of care
- Predischarge patient education
  - ➤ Staff involved
  - ➤ Amount of time
- Role of dietetic technicians
  - ➤ Dietitian—dietetic technician teams
  - ➤ Role expansion to include moderate-risk nutrition assessments and patient education
- Patients' needs
  - ➤ Acuity and length of stay
  - ➤ Time frames for provision of nutrition care
  - ➤ Intensity and frequency of nutrition care
  - ➤ Case management: planning for postdischarge nutrition care

---

neither unit-based procedures nor dietetic technicians are available, the dietitians must complete the nutrition screening themselves. This process can be time-consuming; the screening may divert energy that could be spent caring for nutritionally compromised patients, and it not be the best use of dietitians' knowledge and skills. Using registered dietitians (RDs) for lower-level tasks such as nutrition screening also may contribute to decreased perceptions of their contributions to positive patient outcomes on the part of management staff and members of the health care team.

Some facilities have found the assignment of nutrition screening to unit staff to be problematic because these staff members do not always complete nutrition screening or generate nutrition screening consults according to established policies. The lack of a consistent process for referral of at-risk patients, in addition to being noncompliant with JCAHO standards, may result in the development of backup systems to ensure that (1) RDs have consistent processes for determining daily workload and patient care priorities and (2) at-risk patients receive prompt and thorough nutrition intervention.

The extent of involvement of dietitians in predischarge patient education can have an impact on staffing needs as well. Traditionally, dietitians have provided patient education to meet the JCAHO standard that required education on nutrition, modified diets, and potential nutrient-drug interactions. Because of limited outpatient nutrition services for postdischarge follow-up and the likelihood that patients could not or would not return for follow-up, some dietitians viewed the inpatient stay as a "teachable moment." However, faced with shorter hospital stays, patients who are often too ill or distracted to concentrate on nutrition guidelines, the growing realization that teaching nutrition content and counseling for behavior change are two different activities, and staff reductions, dietitians have streamlined the inpatient education they provide. Now they often provide only "survival skills" information, that is, the information patients need between discharge and their outpatient MNT sessions. For example, the dietitian may review general nutrition guidelines with inpatients with diabetes mellitus and defer an in-depth review of carbohydrate counting to the outpatient setting, when more time is available and patients can concentrate more effectively. Reduced time spent in teaching in the acute setting affects staffing needs, because traditional patient education consumed relatively large blocks of time.

At some facilities, dietetic technicians have assumed responsibility for inpatient nutrition teaching. This enhances their role, and education on survival skills nutrition needs is within the competencies established for dietetic technicians by CADE (10). Provision of basic nutrition education by dietetic technicians allows dietitians' knowledge, skills, and time to be allocated to patients with complex nutrition needs.

In the report on the impact of staffing reductions discussed earlier, Kwon and coauthors noted that most survey respondents reported having increased caseloads (81.3%) and limited time for inpatient diet instruction (84.9%) after cost reductions were made. Ninety percent of respondents reported that they were responsible for nutrition assessment and intervention in high-risk patients, and approximately three fourths reported receiving more high-risk referrals from other health care professionals after cost reductions (5). Although the emphasis on the care of high-risk patients might have been a reflection of the increased acuity of all inpatients observed in recent years, it also might have indicated a reprioritization of the dietitians' time to patients with complex nutrition problems.

Nutrition care activities can affect staffing needs in other ways. For example, when lengths of stay are short and the turnover of patients is frequent, more time will be spent in activities linked to admission (eg, nutrition screening, obtaining food preferences, and initial nutrition assessments).

Certain patient populations require close monitoring and more staff time allocated to monitoring activities. For example, facilities with a high proportion of oncology patients need to accommodate the changing tastes and food tolerances experienced by these patients from day to day, and even from meal to meal. Other patient populations require close monitoring of intake (eg, patients being evaluated for enteral or parenteral nutrition support or for readiness to discontinue this support).

Registered dietitians may spend time in case management activities to promote adherence to postdischarge nutrition care plans. An example of a case management activity is an inpatient dietitian conferring with the dietitian in the patient's postdischarge setting to discuss the patient's nutrition support needs, identify differences in formularies, and select an appropriate substitution. Other examples are arranging delivery of products and supplies through the patient's home health agency and communicating needs for a special infant formula to a local agency of the Special Supplemental Nutrition Program for Women, Infants, and Children (WIC Program).

Another variable that affects staffing needs involves policies established by nutrition departments that specify time frames for the completion of nutrition assessment and reassessment of nutritionally compromised patients and documentation in the medical record. Although no hard and fast rule exists, staff members generally consider both nutritional acuity level and ALOS when determining these time frames. For example, patients who are moderately nutritionally compromised might be assessed within 72 hours of admission, whereas patients considered to be more severely compromised might be assessed within 48 hours of admission. Similarly, reassessment of moderately compromised patients is generally less frequent than that of more severely compromised patients. Staffing needs depend on the numbers of patients at different levels of nutritional risk.

Many nutrition departments have established rescreening policies. In other words, after a defined period, staff members recheck patients who did not have indicators of nutritional risk on admission in order to determine whether these indicators have developed during hospitalization or worsened to the point of needing assessment and intervention. The time frame set for rescreening affects staffing needs, especially if the number of patients needing this activity is high. If the time frame is long (eg, 7 days), many low-risk patients will have been discharged by the time they need rescreening. Conversely, if the time frame is short (eg, 3 days), more patients will still be hospitalized, and a large amount of time may be spent in rescreening.

Documentation

In addition to the time frames established for documenting nutrition care, other factors related to care documentation can affect staffing needs. As mentioned earlier, the use of automation can produce considerable time savings, whereas manual systems may require more staff time. Requirements for documentation of data and results in multiple locations (eg, in both the central medical record and the nutrition department's files) often increase time requirements. The use of checklists, such as interdisciplinary education checklists, usually streamlines documentation.

Teams for Specific Groups of Patients and the Roles and Reporting Relationships of the Staff

In facilities in which teams exist, dietitians are often team members. Roles can vary, and along with this variation comes variation in time commitment to team activities. Dietitians may have small, consultative roles on teams, or they may be very active team members. In some facilities, depending on the type of team, they may even have coordinator roles.

Many facilities admit patients to specific units by service or diagnosis. This strategy promotes the development of specializations and modified team roles for dietitians. They are able to establish collaborative relationships with physicians and members of other disciplines who specialize in working with the patient populations on their units. At these facilities, the dietitians generally follow all patients admitted to their units, not only patients admitted with the diagnoses or conditions in which they specialize.

Some facilities have highly specialized teams or services that follow all team or service patients throughout the facility. In these facilities, team dietitians may follow team patients on units that have assigned dietitians. An issue that often arises is the division of responsibility for nutrition care between the team dietitian and the unit dietitian. Team dietitians may assume total responsibility for the nutrition care of patients being followed by the team, or this responsibility may be shared. Sharing is useful when patients may go off service and the unit dietitians want to be aware of the nutrition care needs of patients who will be reassigned to them. It also ensures continuity of care and appropriate backup coverage when the team dietitian is off.

Staffing needs for the nutrition department are reduced if dietitians on specialized teams cover large numbers of patients and are not members of the nutrition department. However, if these dietitians do not cover many patients or all aspects of their nutrition care (eg, if they cover only nutrition support, not oral diet needs), sufficient nutrition department staff will be needed to ensure adequate coverage. In facilities with this type of cross-coverage, close working relations between team and nonteam registered dietitians are needed to ensure effective communication and optimal nutrition care. On-line documentation and other automated systems facilitate effective communication and seamless patient care.

From a staffing perspective, it might be easier if one RD covered all aspects of nutrition care for patients. However, in a hospital with a career ladder, management of patients' parenteral nutrition may be limited to RDs at the top of the career ladder. An advanced-practice RD might manage the parenteral nutrition for patients on several units, with unit RDs assigned to cover all remaining aspects of their nutrition care. As an example, at Vanderbilt Children's Hospital, a nutrition support dietitian (NSD) who is at the third and highest level of the career ladder, covers parenteral nutrition for all pediatric patients on the nonintensive care units, and unit RDs cover all other aspects of patients' nutrition care. This NSD does not have a unit assignment. In contrast, in the neonatal intensive care and pediatric intensive care units, all aspects of nutrition care, including parenteral nutrition, are managed by the RDs assigned to these units, both of whom are NSDs.

Traditionally, dietitians have been important members of nutrition support teams. However, according to one survey, the number of facilities reporting the presence of nutrition support teams decreased between 1986 and 2000, from 65% of reporting facilities to approximately 50%. In addition, the reported percentage of time spent in nutrition care activities by nutrition support pharmacists in this survey declined from 55% to 30% during the same 14 years (11). In his 2002 presidential address, outgoing president of the American Society for Parenteral and Enteral Nutrition Philip Schneider commented that a similar decrease in time devoted to nutrition support was likely for other members of nutrition support teams as well (12).

These changes are occurring for several likely reasons. Reductions in nutrition support teams have paralleled downsizing initiatives in health care, as teams have been challenged to justify their costs, yet limited in their ability to generate revenues to offset these costs. Reduced time allocation to nutrition support care also might be related to downsizing, as team members find their duties expanded to compensate for reductions in other department staff.

Positive changes in health care that affect the need for nutrition support teams and time allocation for nutrition support care also have occurred. Examples include an increased use of the enteral route for feeding, less overuse of parenteral nutrition support, improved training of health care practitioners who are not nutrition support specialists in the correct provision of nutrition support, availability of nutrition support guidelines and standards of practice, and improved technology to administer and monitor nutrition support (12).

There is evidence that nutrition support teams are effective in reducing the complications of nutrition support, whereas to date, studies have not demonstrated similar positive results in facilities without nutrition support teams. This finding does not necessarily mean that teams are essential, but rather reflects the limited research on the clinical and financial outcomes of teams.

With the focus on patient safety and the specific mention of nutrition support in the AHRQ safety report (13), nutrition managers should pay particular attention to staff competence in nutrition support, adherence to nutrition support guidelines and standards of practice, and selection of nutrition support products that have established efficacy. Both reliance on evidence-based practice and ongoing performance monitoring are essential.

Indirect Care Activities

Indirect care activities are activities that support direct care to patients, including team meetings, patient care rounds, and discharge planning conferences. Involvement of staff in indirect care activities often depends on the amount of time available, and not necessarily on patients' needs. Rounds and team meetings can be very time-consuming and may involve only short discussions of patients' nutrition needs. Dietitians may opt to bypass rounds or team meetings and confer with the

---

Patient Safety and Nutrition Support

When evaluating needs for clinical nutrition staff, consider the impact that nutrition interventions—or in contrast, the lack of interventions—have on patient safety. Factors to consider include the following:

- *Length of time to initiate nutrition interventions.* Is there a delay in identifying the need for nutrition support or the need to discontinue nutrition support?
- *Errors in nutrition support.* Would more registered dietitian hours allow time for more accurate assessment of patients' nutrition needs and time to communicate these needs directly to physicians before orders for nutrition support are written?
- *Changes in patients' status.* Are laboratory values and physical measurements assessed frequently enough and used as a basis for needed alterations in nutrition support?
- *Discharge planning and care.* Are patients adequately prepared for their postdischarge nutrition support care?

physician, nurse, or case manager on a one-to-one basis. Facility and department managers need to define the level of involvement of dietitians in indirect care activities based on required work and availability of staff. They should reach this decision in collaboration with the clinical staff, who can share perspectives about patients' nutrition needs, the value of time spent in teams, and team member perceptions of the value of the dietitians' contributions to team decisions. At some facilities, participation in team rounds and other indirect care activities may be designated for advanced-practice dietitians.

Hours of Operation and Service, Relief, and Weekend Coverage

The staffing plan needs to include adequate staff to cover the hours of operation and service defined in the department scope of services. With recent emphasis by JCAHO on meeting time standards and achieving consistency of care each day of the week, many facilities have increased their weekend staffing. This trend was noted in the survey by Kwon and colleagues; nearly 30% of respondents reported an increase in on-call weekend coverage (5). The responsibility for nutrition screening and the time standards established for direct care activities (eg, assessment of patients at moderate and high risk) determine the need for weekend coverage. This topic will be covered in more detail later in this chapter.

The staffing plan also needs to include coverage for staff who are off during the week and who are on leave for reasons such as vacations, sick leave, and attending professional meetings. Facilities may choose to hire staff whose sole responsibility is relief coverage, or regular staff members may adjust their workloads to accommodate the additional duties of the person who is off. Generally, this method is feasible for an occasional day or a short period of time. However, adequacy of coverage is more difficult when longer time frames are involved.

Scope of Practice and Regulation

Forty-six states have enacted legislation that regulates the practice of dietetics through one of three mechanisms: licensure, statutory certification, or registration. At the time of this writing, 31 states have licensure defining the scope of dietetics practice, 14 states have certification legislation, and 1 state has registration legislation. Regulations that define the role of the dietetic technician are rare. A list of states and the types of practice-related legislation they have is available on the Commission on Dietetic Registration (CDR) Web site (14). This Web site also has links to the Web sites of state regulatory agencies for more in-depth state-by-state information.

Licensure regulations define the scope of dietetic practice and require individuals to obtain licenses prior to performing these activities. Scopes of practice vary from state to state, though the legislation generally includes a definition of dietetics and nutrition practice and lists activities that are examples of practice. Duties and responsibilities assigned to dietitians and dietetic technicians must conform with the scope of practice defined in state licensure laws.

Regulations for statutory certification limit the use of defined titles such as *dietitian, nutritionist,* and *nutrition counselor* to individuals who meet a set of requirements. The regulations do not limit the scope of practice of individuals with certification or of people without certification. Registration is the least restrictive form of legislation related to professional practice and does not limit the scope of practice of professionals.

It is important to consider scope of practice to ensure that roles assigned to dietitians do not exceed any legislated limitations. For example, dietitians may be credentialed to write orders for nutrition support products and laboratory tests to monitor nutrition support. However, they generally cannot order the initiation of nutrition support.

Another example is making a medical diagnosis. Dietitians frequently obtain data that indicate a medical diagnosis, but they are not licensed to make medical diagnoses. In contrast, it is within a dietitian's scope of practice to make nutrition diagnoses and identify nutrition problems. This activity, which is included in the definition of MNT in the Medicare part B MNT legislation, is distinct from medical diagnosing and is an important part of the nutrition care process. Refer to Figure 1.1 for a diagram of the nutrition care process (15).

Patient Care

CMS has defined required nutrition care activities in the conditions of participation for health care facilities. In addition, states have created regulations specific to nutrition care, food safety, and sanitation. These regulations are generally consistent with JCAHO standards, although in some areas, JCAHO standards are more explicit. Copies of the regulations can be obtained from the state health department.

Medicare Part B

In November 2001, Congress passed legislation that defined MNT and provided regulations for the provision of, and billing for, MNT for beneficiaries of the Medicare Part B Program (16). The legislation, which went into effect on January 1, 2002, included the requirement that dietitians provide the MNT benefit, rather than dietetic technicians, registered, dietetic interns, or students; it also required dietitians to become Medicare providers by obtaining provider identification numbers (PINs). PINs are obtained by application to a state Medicare carrier, a company that has contracted with the CMS to manage and pay claims in accordance with Medicare legislation.

The original Medicare Part B MNT legislation established the requirement for reimbursement of dietitians for MNT to be provided by the carriers. However, the CMS has established an alternate billing system for Medicare Part B MNT for use by hospital outpatient billing departments (17). With the alternate system, billing departments can submit claims through another group of CMS contractors, the

> **Definition of Medical Nutrition Therapy**
>
> "Nutritional diagnostic, therapy, and counseling services for the purpose of disease management which are furnished by a registered dietitian or nutrition professional . . . pursuant to a referral by a physician."
>
> —Medicare MNT Benefit, 2002 (16)

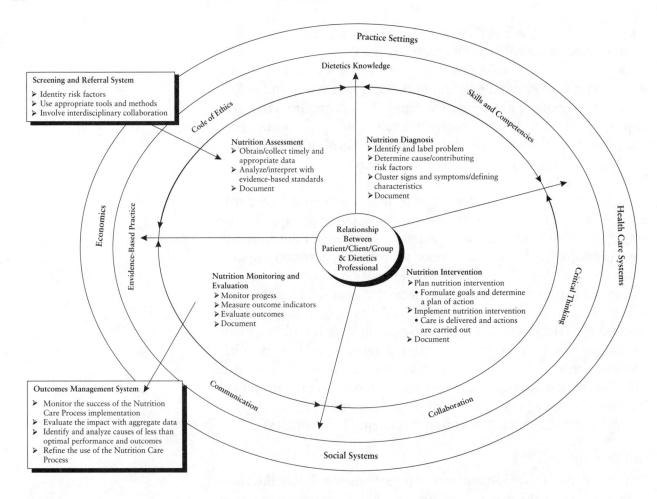

Figure 1.1 ADA Nutrition Care Process and Model. Reprinted from Lacey K. Pritchett E. Nutrition care process and model: ADA adopts road map to quality care and outcomes. *J Am Diet Assoc. 203;103:1061–1072, with permission from the American Dietetic Association.*

Medicare fiscal intermediaries, although PINs are still required for reassignment of benefits to the RDs' employers.

In providing Medicare Part B MNT, dietitians are required to use strict definitions of covered diagnoses, obtain referrals from treating physicians, adhere to national clinical guidelines for assessment and intervention (eg, the *ADA Medical Nutrition Therapy Evidence-Based Guides for Practice* [3]), and keep detailed documentation of the MNT provided and the time spent in face-to-face patient intervention. Dietitians have been authorized to provide MNT without direct physician supervision or even on-site physician oversight, and they can bill Medicare directly for services or assign these benefits to an employer.

This legislation opened up opportunities for dietitians working in outpatient settings and ambulatory clinics to expand their practices. At the same time, it ensured consistency and quality in nutrition intervention by requiring the use of nationally recognized guidelines such as the *ADA Medical Nutrition Therapy Evidence-Based Guides for Practice* (also referred to as *MNT Protocols*). At some facilities, RDs were using the MNT Guides prior to the legislation, although usage data are not available. At other facilities, RDs had to implement the MNT Guides at the same time that other aspects of the new regulations were also being put into place. For these dietitians, implementation resulted in changes in practice ranging from minor to major.

Each MNT Guide defines the number of MNT sessions to be provided for the specified diagnosis and the approximate length of each MNT session. (Refer to the summary page of the type 2 diabetes mellitus MNT Guide in Figure 1.2 [3].) Although the number of sessions and total amounts of time in the protocol may not be identical to those reimbursed via the Medicare Part B benefit, the amounts are similar. The guides clearly specify that MNT be provided in multiple sessions and that monitoring of different types of patient outcomes be done at each session. Examples of outcomes include clinical outcomes such as laboratory data and physical measurements, behavioral outcomes such as nutrient intake and changes in eating habits and patterns, and functional outcomes such as ability to perform activities of daily living and quality of life.

Adequate dietitian time must be allocated to ensure that the MNT Protocols can be implemented and that required documentation can be completed. The total amount of time and the number of staff needed will depend in large part on the number of patients receiving covered services. It is recommended that dietitians follow the same procedures for nutrition care for all patients with the same diagnosis, regardless of the patients' source of payment. Therefore, high volumes of patients with the covered diagnoses will increase the demand for dietitian time, whether MNT is reimbursed by Medicare and non-Medicare third party payers or is paid for by the patients themselves.

It is important to realize that facilities cannot provide MNT for patients covered under the Medicare Part B benefit without complying with the regulations. In other words, RDs cannot provide the service and not charge for it, and they cannot provide the service and ask patients to pay for it out of pocket. Neither practice is allowed, and both put nutrition departments and their facilities in jeopardy of non-compliance with the regulations. An option for facilities that do not want to comply is referral of patients to other facilities where the covered benefit can be obtained. It is also possible for the dietitians to opt out of the program, although the paperwork to do so is very cumbersome, and patients need to be informed of this situation via individual contracts that define their right to obtain the covered service elsewhere.

The members-only section of the ADA Web site (http://www. eatright.org/Member/PolicyInitiatives/83_8722.cfm) has a wealth of resources that provide guidance on implementing the benefit and that link members to relevant Web sites for additional information (18).

Summary Page TYPE 2 DIABETES MELLITUS: *Medical Nutrition Therapy Protocol*

Setting: Ambulatory care or adapted for other health care settings			Number of encounters: 4 to 8 (Grade I)		
No. of encounters	Length of contact	Time between encounters	No. of encounters	Length of contact	Time between encounters
1	60–90 minutes	2–4 weeks	3	30–45 minutes	2–4 weeks
2	30–35 minutes	2–4 weeks	4, 5	30–45 minutes	6–12 months

Expected Outcomes of Medical Nutrition Therapy

Outcome Assessment Factors	Baseline 1	2	3	4	5	Expected Outcomes	Target Goals
Clinical Assessment							
Laboratory Values • Blood glucose	✓	✓	✓	✓	✓	Glucose: ? 10% or at goal	Glucose *Blood mg/dL* *Plasma mg/dL* Preprandial 80–120 90–130 2-hr postprandial 140–160 160–180
• A1C • Lipid profile (fasting cholesterol, HDL-C, LDL-C, TG)	✓ ✓			✓ ✓	✓ ✓	A1C: ↓ by 1 unit or 10% LDL-C: 6%-12% if ≥ 130 HDL-C: ↑ if ≤ 35 TG: ↓ if > 150 mg	A1C: <6% to <7% LDL-C: <100 mg/dL HDL-C: >45 mg/dL, men; >55, women TG: <150 g/dL
• Urine albumin	✓	✓	✓	✓	✓	Urine albumin: ≤ 30 mg/24-h	Urine albumin: Trace
Clinical Signs and Symptoms • Hypo/hyperglycemia • Blood pressure	✓ ✓	✓ ✓	✓ ✓	✓ ✓	✓ ✓	• ↓ hypo/hyperglycemic episodes • Maintains normal blood pressure	• Blood pressure: < 130/80
Nutrition physical • Height • Weight, BMI, Waist Circumference						• Maintains healthy weight and appropriate waist circumference • Men: < 102 cm (< 40 inches) • Women: < 88 cm (< 35 inches)	• If > 25, a 5%-10% decrease (Grade II)
Therapeutic/Lifestyle Changes*							**MNT Goal**
• Food/meal planning	✓	✓	✓	✓	✓	• Chooses meals/snacks from a variety of foods, including fruits, vegetables, grains, cereals, dairy products • Eats meals/snacks at appropriate times • Chooses food and amounts per meal pattern • Energy intake to meet glucose/weight loss goals • Adjusts protein intake for weight control and to prevent complications • ↓ fat to improve serum lipids and improve insulin sensitivity • Distributes carbohydrate to achieve glucose goals; adjusts carbohydrates to achieve glucose/TG goals • Limits foods ↑ in sodium	• Adheres to meal plan, exercise and medication treatment plan to achieve blood glucose and lipid goals • ↓ kcal 250–500 of usual intake for gradual weight ↓ • Protein: 15%-20% of daily energy intake if renal function normal. Limit protein to 0.8–1.0 g/kg with nephropathy (Grade II) • Fat: percentage of kcal from total fat: 25%–35%, < 7% SF, 10% PUFA, 10%–15% MUFA, < 200 mg cholesterol (Grade I) • Carbohydrate: > 45% kcal; consistency (Grade I) • < 2,400 mg/day
• Food preparation	✓					• Uses cooking techniques to modify fat/kcal/sodium intake	
• Recipe modification			✓			• Modifies recipes as needed	
• Food label reading		✓				• Accurately reads food labels	
• Dining out			✓			• Selects appropriate foods	
• Physical activity	✓	✓	✓	✓	✓	• Participates in aerobic activity to achieve blood glucose and weight goals (Grade II)	• 3–4 × per week, 30–60 minutes/day (burn a minimum of 1,500 kcal per week)
• Self-monitoring of blood glucose	✓	✓	✓	✓	✓	• Daily records: food/glucose/physical activity; adjusts food/physical activity to meet glucose goals • Uses insulin or sulfonylureas to decrease blood glucose	• Check blood glucose 4 ×/day (Grade IV)
• Knowledge of signs and symptoms, prevention and treatment of hypo/hyperglycemia	✓	✓				• Recognizes signs and symptoms of hyper- and hypoglycemia	
• Sick day management		✓				• Modifies food selection and eating schedule	• Check blood glucose and ketones more frequently
• Smoking cessation						• Verbalizes importance of smoking cessation	
• Alcohol use						• Limits alcohol use to < 2 drinks per day for men and < 1 drink per day for women	
• Knowledge of potential food/drug interaction	✓	✓	✓	✓	✓	• Verbalizes potential food/drug interaction	

*Encounter in which behavioral topics are covered may vary according to client's readiness, skills, resources, and need for lifestyle changes.

Figure 1.2 Summary page, Type 2 diabetes mellitus: medical nutrition therapy protocol. Reprinted with permission from Nutrition practice guidelines type 2 diabetes mellitus. *American Dietetic Association Medical Nutrition Therapy Evidence-Based Guides for Practice* [CD-ROM]. © 2001, American Dietetic Association

Accreditation Standards, Procedures, and Audits

In health care, most facilities use the standards published by JCAHO (19). These standards provide a framework for facility operations and define the processes that must be used in developing, implementing, and evaluating patient care. Operational standards apply to all departments of the facility, including the nutrition department, unless otherwise stated.

In 2004, JCAHO launched a new accreditation process, which is described in detail in Appendix A. In preparation for the launch of the new process, JCAHO created a Standards Review Task Force to identify standards that could be deleted, consolidated with other standards, or reorganized. The goal of this review was to focus standards on those processes that are critical to patient safety and the quality of care. To promote understanding of the consolidated 2004 standards, JCAHO published crosswalks for each chapter of each accreditation manual, linking the 2004 standards with the standards in the 2003 accreditation manual. The new standards differ in format from the earlier ones. The new format includes an overview of each chapter, the standards, and the elements of performance (EP) that are subject to review by JCAHO surveyors, with surveyor assessment and scoring protocols. To promote consistency in the survey process, each standard clearly communicates the requirements for compliance. Some standards have a rationale that defines the purpose of the standard.

A review of all relevant sections of the accreditation manual, the standards, and the EP is recommended to obtain specific and detailed information. It is also recommended that any questions about facility-specific implementation of standards be clarified directly with JCAHO staff.

Nutrition Care

The standards relevant to patient care have been consolidated into one section of the accreditation manual, "Provision of Care, Treatment, and Services" (PC). The overview for this section of the manual describes a cyclical process for patient care that is individualized, interdisciplinary, collaborative, and coordinated within the facility and with external facilities providing care to the patient. For nutrition, the cyclical process originates with nutrition screening to identify characteristics associated with malnutrition or the risk of malnutrition. When the characteristics of malnutrition or the risk of malnutrition is identified, nutrition screening is followed by nutrition assessment and the development of a plan for nutrition care, implementation of the nutrition interventions defined in the care plan, and monitoring of the patient's response to nutrition care.

According to the EP, nutrition screening must be completed within 24 hours of admission to an inpatient facility, and the facility should have a seamless process for nutrition assessment of patients determined to be at nutritional risk. JCAHO allows for preadmission completion of nutrition screening, as long as completion occurs not more than 30 days prior to admission and any changes that occur between preadmission completion and actual admission are documented in the medical record on admission.

Under these umbrella standards, JCAHO requires each facility to define its policies and procedures for nutrition screening, nutrition assessment, and reassessment. Although JCAHO does not describe specific requirements for the content of nutrition assessments or time frames for completion, facility policies and procedures do need to define them. JCAHO does define the general elements of an assessment: collecting data; analyzing data to produce information about a patient's needs and to identify the need for additional data; and making care, treatment, or service decisions based on the information about a patient's needs and response to care, treatment, and services.

The facility should individualize the plan of care according to the patient's needs; involve the patient in the plan's development to the greatest extent possible; include care goals that are reasonable and measurable; and include regular review and revision based on the patient's response to care, treatment, and services. The use of the Nutrition Care Process and Model that is described later in this chapter ensures that RDs will be successful in implementing the standards in the "Provision of Care, Treatment, and Services" section of the accreditation manual.

Patients should be educated about their care and treatment, in order to participate in the decision-making process and to take responsibility for self-management activities. As appropriate, this patient education includes education about nutrition interventions and modified diets.

Food and nutrition products are to be provided for the patient as appropriate to care, treatment, and services. This provision includes honoring patients' cultural, religious, and ethnic food preferences; offering substitute foods of equal nutritional value when patients refuse to eat the food that is served; appropriately storing food brought in by patients; and accommodating special diets and altered diet schedules.

Impact. As noted earlier, facilities vary in the procedures they choose to implement the standards and their EP. The extent of variation makes interfacility comparisons and benchmarking more difficult. This variation also contributes to difficulty in collecting and evaluating data related to the impact of staffing changes on the outcomes of nutrition intervention. Several examples of variation were discussed previously.

Another way that facilities vary is in the criteria selected to define nutritional risk. Ideally, the criteria selected are evidence based, are able to accurately identify patients with nutrition problems, and are applied to all patients. However, it is likely that many facilities have not assessed the validity or reliability of their nutrition screening processes.

At many facilities, patients at nutritional risk are further subdivided according to the severity of their nutrition problems. Categorization of patients into different levels of nutritional risk serves two purposes. First, it allows determination of patients' nutritional status and their degree of nutritional impairment, based on comparison of nutritional risk criteria and other relevant data with norms and standards. Second, as noted earlier, it provides input for a system of prioritization of patients and their nutrition needs that results in daily work assignments of staff. In other words, the system helps staff members know what work they have to do each day.

At some facilities, patients are divided into two nutritional risk categories: patients who are at risk and those who are not at risk. At many facilities, however, nutritionally compromised patients are divided into three, and sometimes four, levels (eg, low, moderate, and high nutritional risk levels or low, moderate, high, and very high nutritional risk levels). Table 1.1 provides an example of a system for determining nutritional risk categories for adult patients (20). Box 1.2 provides an example of a system for pediatric patients (9).

The Department of Veterans Affairs (VA) health care system has developed a comprehensive system for nutrition screening and categorization of nutritional risk (20). The VA patient classification system classifies inpatients into 18 care categories based on nutritional status, bed section, and length of stay; it classifies outpatients into 8 outpatient groups based on type of nutrition care (ie, education versus intervention), visit type (ie, new patient or follow-up), and medical center type. The classification system, reported in the July 2001 issue of the *Journal of the American Dietetic Association,* has been rigorously evaluated for its validity and reliability within the VA health care system and is available, with instructions for its use, on the Internet at http://*www.hsrd.ann-arbor.med.va.gov/clinutstaf_jcl.htm* (21). It is a model for facilities to use in developing their own system, although validity and reliability need to be established on a facility-by-facility basis.

Methods of collecting data for nutrition screening and assessment also contribute to variation. Patients provide historical data about their weight and intake histories, appetite and appetite changes, and other signs and symptoms of their problems. These subjective data are used along with objective data, such as weight and height, to identify nutritional risk. Many facilities use self-reported weights and heights. Others weigh patients but use self-reported heights. The use of estimated weights poses problems in identifying subtle weight changes. The use of estimated heights can affect the accuracy of comparisons of actual weights with ideal weights, if ideal weights are calculated using heights.

Another example of variation in the implementation of the JCAHO standards is the selection of time frames to complete nutrition assessments and reassessments. Patients with greater nutrition needs should receive nutrition assessment and nutrition care plans more rapidly than patients with lower-priority needs, and patients at higher risk

Table 1.1 Nutrition Care Level Evaluation Criteria—Adults*

Category	1 Point	2 Points	3 Points	4 Points	Highest Ratings (Check 3)
Nutrition history	• Good appetite • Eating/digestion problems, none • Independent ADL	• Fair appetite • Chewing problems • Constipation • Limited ADL • Nausea • Requires feeding assistance • Restricted ambulation	• Poor appetite • Diarrhea • Swallowing problems • Vomiting	• No appetite	
Albumin (nondilutional)—metabolic stress	= 3.5 g/dL	3.0–3.4 g/dL	2.5–2.9 g/dL	< 2.4 g/dL	
Diagnosis (examples from full list)	• Total hip replacement • Hypertension • Electrolyte imbalance	• Cardiac disease • Stable COPD • CVA • Controlled diabetes • Pneumonia	• Head and neck cancer • CHF • Stage III pressure ulcer • New spinal cord injury	• Acute renal failure • Bone marrow transplant • Malnutrition • Multiple trauma	
Weight history (unintentional loss as % of IBW)	Stable, no loss	< 10% in 6 mo	10%–15% in 6 mo or < 7.5% in 3 mo or < 5% in 1 mo or < 2% in 1 wk	> 15% in 6 mo or > 7.5% in 3 mo or > 5% in 1 mo or > 2% in 1 week	
Weight status (current weight as % of IBW)	90%–100% IBW or < 119% IBW	81%–89% IBW or 120%–129% IBW	75%–80% IBW or 130%–149% IBW	< 74% IBW or > 150% IBW	
Current diet order	• Regular • Mechanical	• Diabetic/weight reduction • Consistency modified, except mechanical • Drug-nutrient interaction • Dysphagia • Lactose-free • Low fat/low cholesterol • Sodium restricted	• Fluid restricted (<1,000 mL) • Mineral restricted, other than sodium • Protein restricted • Tube feeding, stable	• Clear liquid > 3 d • NPO > 3 d • Parenteral nutrition support • Tube feeding—new or unstable	Total points from 3 categories with highest ratings

Abbreviations: ADL, activities of daily living; COPD, chronic obstructive pulmonary disease; CVA, cerebrovascular accident; CHF, congestive heart failure; IBW, ideal body weight; NPO, nothing by mouth.

*In use at Vanderbilt University Medical Center.

Source: Adapted from Hiller L, Lowery JC, Davis JA, Shore CJ, Striplin DT. Nutritional status classification in the Department of Veterans Affairs. *J Am Diet Assoc.* 2001;101:786–792, with permission from the American Dietetic Association.

Nutrition Risk Category:

(Add scores for the 3 categories with the most points. Must have scores for 4 of 6 categories.)

Low (3–5 points) _____   Moderate (6–8 points) _____   High (9–11 points) _____   Very high (= 12 points) _____

Box 1.2 Vanderbilt Children's Hospital Nutrition Risk Evaluation Criteria for Infants and Children

I. **Nutrient Intake**—1 point for each of the following:
Severe nausea and/or vomiting (= 3 days), and/or diarrhea (> 500 mL × 2 days)
Reduced food intake > 5 days (< 66% of usual amount)
Potential for prolonged poor intake

II. **Albumin (nondilutional)**
3.2–3.4 g/dL (1 point)   2.8–3.1 g/dL (2 points)
2.4–2.7 g/dL (3 points)   2.3 g/dL or below (4 points)

III. **Increased Metabolic Requirements**
Surgery since admission (1 point)

IV. **Growth History**
Unintentional weight loss in past 12 months (2 points)
Poor/excessive weight gain (2 points):
- Weight for height/length < 10th percentile or > 90th percentile
- Weight for age < 5th percentile or > 95th percentile
- Height for age < 5th percentile

V. **Modified Diet (1 point) and/or Food Allergy (1 point)**

Points and Preliminary Plan of Care:
0–1 point = Nutrition assessment indicated—Evaluate learning needs; rescreen after 5 days.
2–3 points = Nutrition assessment indicated within 72 hours of admission; reassess at least weekly.
4 or more points or Nutrition Support or Special/concentrated infant formula = Nutrition assessment indicated within 48 hours of admission; reassess twice weekly.

Source: Adapted with permission from Pediatric Nutrition Care Level Evaluation Process used at Vanderbilt University Medical Center (9).

---

levels should have more frequent monitoring and reassessment than patients at lower risk levels.

The time frames selected have a large impact on staffing requirements. For example, if a facility specifies that high nutritional risk assessments for newly admitted patients are to be completed within 48 hours of admission, both the volume of patients admitted at high nutritional risk and the overall facility admission patterns will affect staffing requirements. Elective admissions generally occur on weekdays. Non-elective admissions occur at any time, although clusters can be observed in some facilities (eg, more trauma admissions may occur on weekends and holidays because of an increase in motor vehicle accidents and gunshot wounds). With a time standard for completion of high nutritional risk assessments within 48 hours of admission, weekend dietitian staffing is needed to ensure that this time frame can be met.

JCAHO standards apply to emergency departments, ambulatory clinics, and other affiliated outpatient practices. Implementation of JCAHO standards in these settings, especially standards for nutrition screening, has proved to be a challenge at some facilities.

JCAHO recently released a publication to assist facilities in their compliance with the standards for patient care (22). In addition to clarifying the standards and intent statements, the publication includes numerous examples of nutrition screening and assessment programs and the forms used by facilities to meet JCAHO standards.

Human Resources Standards

In 2002, JCAHO revised its human resources (HR) standards as a result of concern about the nationwide shortage of health care workers (especially the shortage of nurses), the reduction in enrollment in training programs for all health professions, and the aging of the nurse and health care provider workforce. JCAHO considers staffing shortages to be a threat to patient safety; it cites as evidence the documentation of insufficient staffing level as a factor in a sizable number of reported sentinel events. JCAHO also states that likely results of inadequate staffing include reductions in the quality of patient care and in the ability of hospitals to respond to mass casualties.

In the "Overview" section of the 2004 HR standards, JCAHO describes the outcome or goal to be achieved through the implementation of the standards: the identification and provision of the "right number of competent staff to meet the patients' needs" (19). The overview and standards expand on this goal by describing four processes that managers should carry out.

The first process is providing an adequate number of staff to fulfill the facility's mission and meet the needs of populations receiving care and services. Managers are expected to define projected needs and compare their projections with data on actual staffing and staff qualifications, using variances to support requests for additional staff or refine qualifications. In defining qualifications needed for positions, managers are expected to comply with legal and regulatory requirements, as well as with hospital policies.

Facilities are required to evaluate the effectiveness of their staffing by selecting at least four screening indicators to measure and analyze, using a specified rationale for their indicator selection. They also are required to define expected performance; a method or methods for data collection, analysis, and reporting; and the direct and indirect caregivers whose level of staffing could affect each indicator. Two of the indicators selected must be clinical/service indicators and the other two, HR indicators. Furthermore, one indicator from each category must be selected from a JCAHO-identified screening indicator list. Examples of clinical/service indicators on the JCAHO-identified list are patient complaints, family complaints, skin breakdown, pneumonia, postoperative infections, and adverse drug events. Examples of JCAHO-identified HR indicators are amount of overtime, staff vacancy rate, staff turnover rate, sick time use, staff satisfaction, and understaffing identified by comparison with the staffing plan.

JCAHO has been careful to explain to accredited facilities that it is not necessary to collect indicator data for departments in which staff members are not involved directly or indirectly in patient care (eg, the marketing or accounts payable departments). Individual departments with staff who are identified as either direct or indirect care providers that affect the screening indicators selected are not expected to collect their own data independently, but rather are expected to participate in facility-wide efforts.

It is likely that nutrition department staff, including dietitians, dietetic technicians, and support staff (eg, diet aides and tray delivery staff), may be identified by a facility as care providers whose staffing affects indicator performance. When this is the case, managers and staff will participate in data collection, analysis, and reporting, as well as in PI initiatives.

As an example, a facility that selected the clinical/service indicators of pneumonia rate and urinary tract infection (UTI) rate and the HR indicators of staff turnover rate and staff satisfaction might discover that a high rate of turnover among nutrition department staff assigned to deliver and pick up patient trays was a factor in decreased job satisfaction among nurses on specific units. This decreased satisfaction might result from their having to assume more nonclinical duties, such as tray delivery and pickup. A more in-depth analysis of the data in combination might show that on the units with higher turnover in nursing staff, rates of pneumonia and UTI were also higher. A PI plan to address rates of pneumonia and UTIs would need to examine nursing satisfaction and turnover, as well as turnover of the nutrition department staff who deliver and pick up patient trays. This example illustrates the interrelationships that exist among staff of departments in a facility and how factors in one area can affect performance in another, to the extent of producing negative patient outcomes.

Outpatient clinics were not expected to evaluate staffing effectiveness. However, JCAHO is planning to expand the collection of indicator data in outpatient clinics affiliated with accredited organizations.

The second process that managers should carry out is providing competent staff and confirming competency initially and during orientation by verifying licenses, certifications, and registrations. Verification can occur through several mechanisms—for example, viewing an original license or a renewal certificate and keeping a copy of the document in the employee's file; checking an on-line database of active licenses or credentialed professionals maintained by the licensing or credentialing board; or sending a letter to the board when an individual has lost the certificate and the board does not maintain an on-line database of active licenses. A record of verification of all credentials should be maintained in employee files (23).

JCAHO–Screening Indicators for Hospitals

Human Resources
- Sick time
- Nursing care time per patient day
- On-call or per diem use
- Overtime
- Staff injuries
- Staff satisfaction
- Staff turnover rate
- Staff vacancy rate
- Understaffing compared with the staffing plan

Clinical/Service
- Adverse drug events
- Falls
- Injuries to patients
- Length of stay
- Patient complaints
- Family complaints
- Pneumonia
- Postoperative infections
- Skin breakdown (pressure ulcers)
- Shock/cardiac arrest
- Upper gastrointestinal tract bleeding
- Urinary tract infections

Source: Adapted from *2003 Hospital Accreditation Standards: Tools for Performance Measurement in Health Care: A Quick Reference Guide.* Oakbrook Terrace, Ill: Joint Commission Resources; 2002:246–247, with permission from Joint Commission Resources.

Assessing Staff Competency

The process of assessing staff competency begins with recruitment and continues throughout employment:

- **Recruitment** of applicants using the requirements and competencies listed on the job description. *Be sure that the education and training requirements and the knowledge, skills, and competencies of positions have been explained thoroughly to the human resources recruiter.*
- **Initial assessment** of applicants' credentials and qualifications.
- **Orientation** confirmation of the experience, education, and abilities of newly hired staff members.
- **Ongoing competency assessment** conducted throughout employment at intervals defined by the facility to evaluate staff members' continuing abilities to perform their duties and responsibilities.

The third process that managers should carry out is orienting, training, and educating staff through ongoing programs specific to work-related issues. And the fourth process is assessing, improving, and maintaining staff competence to ensure continuing ability of staff to perform their duties and responsibilities.

An example of an identified learning need is the need for additional knowledge and skills related to the selection of appropriate nutrition support and the methods for monitoring patients' tolerance of their nutrition support. This need could be identified in a variety of ways (eg, through peer review, self-assessment, or evaluation of department PI data). In this example, additional training and skill building can be achieved through attendance at a national or regional nutrition support seminar, professional self-study using on-line materials available through the American Society for Parenteral and Enteral Nutrition, and peer-to-peer training by a certified nutrition support dietitian.

Impact. To comply with the HR standards, nutrition managers must evaluate their staffing needs in a systematic manner, and they must participate in facility-wide efforts to evaluate staffing effectiveness. The information in this book can be used to complete an evaluation of staffing needs and to justify levels of staffing provided or requested. In addition, adequate time must be allocated for the orientation, training, and ongoing education of staff to ensure a competent and qualified workforce. The topic of staffing effectiveness is discussed in more detail in Chapter 6.

Performance Improvement Standards

JCAHO has defined the components of PI as measuring performance through data collection, assessing current performance, and improving performance. The goal is a reduction in factors leading to unanticipated adverse events or outcomes. Facility-wide priorities for PI must be established in a planned, systematic, and organization-wide approach that ensures collaboration among services (19).

Use of evidence-based clinical practice guidelines is a method suggested by JCAHO to reduce undesirable variation in patient care processes. Guidelines can assist practitioners in improving the appropriate use and effectiveness of health care services and in reducing the risk of errors, therefore contributing to improved patient safety.

Impact. Adequate staffing must be available to support facility and department PI initiatives and activities. RDs are encouraged to use the *ADA Medical Nutrition Therapy Evidence-Based Guides for Practice* (3) to reduce practice variation and improve the quality of nutrition care provided.

Professional Accountabilities

The information in this section has a different emphasis than the information included in the first four areas. The information in these areas defined considerations that were external in their origin—that is, information gleaned from completing an organizational and departmental scan and a review of the regulations and standards that must be followed to meet legal requirements, receive payment for services, and achieve accreditation.

The information in the fifth area covers the accountabilities that dietitians and dietetic technicians have because they are members of a profession that is committed to enhancing the nutritional well-being of people. The focus is internal—specific to the profession of dietetics. The accountabilities are shared by each nutrition department as a unit and by the individual members of each department as dietetics professionals.

Code of Ethics

The American Dietetic Association (ADA) and its Commission on Dietetic Registration have adopted a voluntary, enforceable code of ethics entitled the Code of Ethics for the Profession of Dietetics. (24) The code can be accessed in its entirety on the ADA Web site at http://www.eatright.org/Member/Governance/index_18917.cfm (25). The purpose of the code is to guide dietetics professionals in their professional practice and conduct.

The entire code applies to members of ADA who are RDs and dietetic technicians, registered. The code also applies to all ADA members who are not RDs or dietetic technicians, registered, except for the items specific to credentialing, and to RDs and dietetic technicians, registered, who are not members of ADA, except for the items specific to ADA membership.

The code consists of a set of 19 principles. Some of the principles are broad in scope (eg, conducting oneself with honesty, integrity, and fairness). Others define how the work of dietetics is to be done. For example, practice is to be based on scientific information and current information. Information should be presented to clients without bias and in a manner that promotes informed decision making, with sensitivity to cultural differences and without discrimination. Although the overwhelming majority of dietitians and dietetic technicians undoubtedly would agree that they practice according to the code, the importance of doing so cannot be overstated. In developing a staffing plan, consideration should be given to following each principle defined in the code.

Standards of Professional Practice

In addition to the Code of Ethics, ADA has adopted standards that provide more specific guidance about how dietetic practice is to be conducted: the Standards of Professional Practice, or SOPP (26). The SOPP apply to all areas of practice and dietetics professionals, and they define the minimum level of performance expected. Each standard is presented in a format that includes the standard statement, its rationale, indicators for performance, and examples of outcomes. The SOPP can be accessed in their entirety on the ADA Web site at *http://www.eatright.com/qm/standardslist.html* (27). The standard for application of research, "effectively applies, participates in or generates research to enhance practice," reinforces the importance of translating research findings into dietetic practice. An example of the translation of research into practice is the routine implementation of the *ADA Medical Nutrition Therapy Evidence-Based Guides for Practice* (3) by outpatient dietitians. This practice includes the consistent monitoring of outcomes for individual clients and the use of aggregate outcomes for groups of patients with the same diagnosis, in order to improve overall department performance. The performance standard for the dietitian is the understanding and use of the MNT Guides. The staffing plan for an outpatient clinic must allow adequate time for this practice to occur.

Two standards, those for the utilization and management of resources and for quality in practice, have particular relevance to planning, implementing, and evaluating staffing and a staffing plan (see Boxes 1.3 and 1.4) (27). The following SOPP have been developed for specific subsets of dietetics professionals:

- *National Standards for Diabetes Self-Management Education*, Diabetes Task Force (*Diabetes Care.* 1995;95[suppl 1]:94–96). An updated description of the roles of RD, RD/certified diabetes educator, and dietetic technician, registered, is available in the October 2000 *Journal of the American Dietetic Association.* (28)
- *Standards of Practice for the Consultant Dietitian*, Consultant Dietitians in Health Care Facilities DPG (*J Am Diet Assoc.* 1993;93:305–308).
- *Standards of Practice Criteria for Clinical Nutrition Managers*, Clinical Nutrition Management DPG (*J Am Diet Assoc.* 1997;97:673–678).
- *Standards of Practice for Gerontological Nutritionists: A Mandate for Action*, Gerontological Nutritionists DPG (*J Am Diet Assoc.* 1995;95:1433–1438).
- *Standards of Practice for the Nutrition Support Dietitian*, Dietitians in Nutrition Support DPG—a joint project with the American Society for Parenteral and Enteral Nutrition (ASPEN) (*J Am Diet Assoc.* 1993;93:1113–1116). The most current revision of the standards of practice can be accessed on the ASPEN Web site under standards of practice (http://*www.nutritioncare.org/profdev/rdstandards.pdf.*) (29).

Practice Audit

The CDR has conducted practice audits at periodic intervals since 1989 to profile the work that dietitians and dietetic technicians actually perform. The most recent update of audit data was completed in 1999 and published in 2000 (30). The 1999 audit included three components: (1) a survey of entry-level and beyond-entry-level dietitians

---

Box 1.3   Standard 4: Utilization and Management of Resources

Uses resources effectively and efficiently in practice

Rationale

Appropriate use of time, money, facilities, and human resources facilitates delivery of quality services.

Indicators—Each dietetics professional:

4.1 uses a systematic approach to maintain and manage professional resources successfully

4.2 uses measurable resources such as personnel, monies, equipment, guidelines, protocols, reference materials, and time in the provision of dietetics services

4.3 analyzes safety, effectiveness, and cost in planning and delivering services and products

4.4 justifies use of resources by documenting consistency with plan, continuous quality improvement, and desired outcomes

4.5 educates and helps clients and others to identify and secure appropriate and available resources and services

Examples of outcomes

- The dietetics professional documents use of resources according to plan and budget.
- Resources and services are measured and data are used to promote and validate the effectiveness of services.
- Desired outcomes are achieved and documented.
- Resources are managed and used cost-effectively.

Source: Reprinted with permission from Standards of professional practice. American Dietetic Association Web site. Available at: http://www.eatright.org/Member/83_9468.cfm. Accessed February 6, 2004.

---

and dietetic technicians, to learn the duties and responsibilities in their current positions and their anticipated performance of a subset of duties; (2) a survey of a parallel sample of employers to learn about actual and anticipated duties of dietitians and dietetic technicians; and (3) focus group discussions with employers to identify their perceptions of emerging roles for dietetics professionals and the competencies needed to support these roles.

The 1999 audit provides a valuable resource for use in developing staffing plans, because it defines in detail the duties that dietitians and dietetic technicians complete in their work in health care settings. The data also permit benchmarking—that is, the comparison of actual or proposed staff duties and responsibilities with those being completed by other dietetics professionals and with the perceived needs of their employers.

Of note is the fact that the 1999 data from both dietitians and employers indicate stability in roles since the 1989 audit. Dietitians in

Box 1.4   Standard 5: Quality in Practice

Systematically evaluates the quality and effectiveness of practice and revises practice as needed to incorporate the results of evaluation

Rationale
Quality practice requires regular performance evaluation and continuous improvement of services.

Indicators—Each dietetics professional:
5.1 identifies performance improvement criteria to monitor effectiveness of services
5.2 identifies expected outcomes
5.3 documents outcomes of services provided
5.4 compares actual performance to expected outcomes
5.5 documents action taken when discrepancies exist between actual performance and expected outcomes
5.6 continuously evaluates and refines services based on measured outcomes

Examples of outcomes
- Performance improvement criteria are measured.
- Actual performance is evaluated.
- Clients' outcomes meet established criteria (objectives/goals).
- Results of quality improvement activities direct refinement of practice.

Source: Reprinted with permission from Standards of professional practice. American Dietetic Association Web site. Available at: http://www.eatright.org/Member/83_9468.cfm. Accessed February 6, 2004.

the 1999 audit report being more involved in requesting laboratory tests and collecting data than in the earlier audit, as well as being less involved in performing anthropometric measurements. Otherwise, no substantial differences were found between their roles in 1989 and 1999.

Although this finding can be considered in a positive light (ie, roles have not diminished and are not expected to do so), much changed in health care between 1989 and 1999. It might be theorized that dietitians did not redefine their roles to keep pace with these changes, either out of choice or because they were not allowed to do so. For more information on future practice roles, see Chapter 2.

Components of Dietetic Practice

During the early 1990s, the CDR conducted research using a Delphi procedure to identify the components of dietetic practice. The research identified 21 practice components. These components served as the foundation for the development of nine self-assessment modules that dietitians and dietetic technicians can use to assess and develop their competencies in specific areas of practice. Specific competencies were defined for each module. A list of these competencies can be found in Appendix C of the ADA publication *Ensuring Staff Competence* (31).

In addition, while developing the test specifications for board certification for specialization in renal, pediatric, and metabolic nutrition practice, the CDR defined specialty-specific practice competencies based on the results of role delineation studies and practice audits. The full list of competency domains and competencies also can be found in Appendix C of *Ensuring Staff Competence* (31). Information on ordering the self-assessment modules and the specialty practice self-assessment simulations is available from the ADA Web site or the ADA Products and Services Catalog.

Job Descriptions and Competencies

Job descriptions define position requirements, competencies, and duties and responsibilities. They are used in hiring, orienting, and evaluating performance of staff. HR departments also use job descriptions to determine appropriate staff compensation and ensure internal pay equity among different types of staff. To do so, HR staff members review job descriptions for what are known as *compensable factors*. Points or weights are given for all factors identified, and final ratings and pay grades of positions are assigned based on the total number of points given to the job descriptions. To ensure accurate evaluation, job descriptions should list duties and responsibilities in descending order of importance. They also should describe the complexity of decision making, the skill sets required, accountabilities, contacts, and minimum requirements (32).

Another method of determining compensation often favored by HR staff involves the external market model, which uses salary comparisons of average current pay for positions being evaluated. Both regional averages and averages for similar-sized facilities are used for comparison. However, salary averages may not reflect differences in duties and responsibilities of staff or differences in patients' nutritional acuity (ie, the nutrition case mix) among the comparison facilities. Therefore, careful matching with comparison facilities is important. The results of external comparisons can be used to support salary adjustments to maintain market competitiveness (32).

Like staffing plans, job descriptions need to be reviewed regularly and updated as needed to reflect changes made in position requirements and in duties and responsibilities. ADA has published a valuable resource on job descriptions, *Job Descriptions: Models for Dietetics Profession* (33). This publication includes actual job descriptions for dietitians and dietetic technicians who work in all practice settings and who have many different types of duties and levels of responsibility.

Impact. The competencies described above can be used to compare the roles defined for clinical nutrition staff with the roles identified by the CDR. Variance from these competencies can serve as an impetus for refining and enhancing roles and for updating job descriptions.

Self-Assessment Series for Dietetics Professionals

The following titles are available from the American Dietetic Association (http://www.eatright.org/catalog or 800/877-1600 ext. 5000):

- *Nutrition Assessment*
- *Nutrition Care Planning*
- *Implementing Nutrition Care*
- *Evaluating Nutrition Care Plans*
- *Nutrition Counseling*
- *Nutrition Education for Consumers*
- *Research in Practice*
- *Management*
- *Marketing Products, Services, and Yourself*

Nutrition Care Process and Model

The past few years have witnessed an evolving awareness of the need for a consistent process for delivering nutrition care to individual patients and groups of patients that is recognized by the dietetics profession (ie, officially approved by the ADA House of Delegates). This need grew from an increasing recognition of the variation in practice among dietitians and dietetic technicians—variation that potentially has limited the positive impact of nutrition intervention. In addition, the lack of a model for providing nutrition care has contributed to the difficulty experienced within the profession in conducting research to document the impact of nutrition care on health care outcomes. The need was confirmed by the realization that other health care professions (eg, nursing, physical therapy, and occupational therapy) have developed and implemented their own care processes.

In 2002, the Quality Management Committee of the House of Delegates appointed the Nutrition Care Process Workgroup and charged it with developing a draft Nutrition Care Process in time for consideration at the Fall 2002 ADA House of Delegates meeting. The group met during the summer of 2002 to develop options of models for a process. In preparation, the work group reviewed several models of processes that had been published in the professional literature and used by dietetic educators to train students and interns. The final Nutrition Care Process and Model was approved by the House of Delegates in May 2003 and published in the August *Journal of the American Dietetic Association* (15). Figure 1.1 contains a diagram of the model. Figure 1.3 illustrates a practical use for the model (15).

Impact. Use of the Nutrition Care Process and Model has implications for clinical nutrition staffing. First, its adoption by the ADA House of Delegates made it imperative that dietitians and dietetic technicians in all settings review their practices to ensure application of the process in its entirety. In addition, managers must allocate sufficient time in their clinical nutrition staffing plans for the process to be used. One activity required to assess staffing needs is measuring time allocations for different types of nutrition intervention and for patients at different levels of nutritional risk (described in detail in Chapter 3). As dietetic practice evolves over the next few years through implementation of the Nutrition Care Process, periodic remeasurements of time allocations will be essential to ensure accurate predictions of staffing needs.

Medical Nutrition Therapy Guides for Practice and Protocols

The first MNT Protocols were published by ADA in 1996 (34). The following year additional protocols were published (35), and in 1998 the original protocols were revised (36). The Quality Management Committee of ADA, which oversees the development of all protocols and other practice guides, created a definition of MNT Protocols to enhance understanding of their importance to dietetic practice. According to this definition, each MNT Protocol is a plan or set of

---

The Nutrition Care Process

During nutrition assessment, data are obtained and compared with existing norms and standards. This activity results in the identification of actual or potential nutritional deficits or excesses that are stated as nutrition diagnoses or problems. The signs and symptoms that indicate a nutrition diagnosis or problem are also defined, along with actual or presumed etiologies. Nutrition interventions are selected based on their ability to alter the etiologies or causes of the problems. The goal of nutrition intervention is normalization of, or improvement in, the original signs and symptoms, which is determined through monitoring and reassessment at defined intervals.

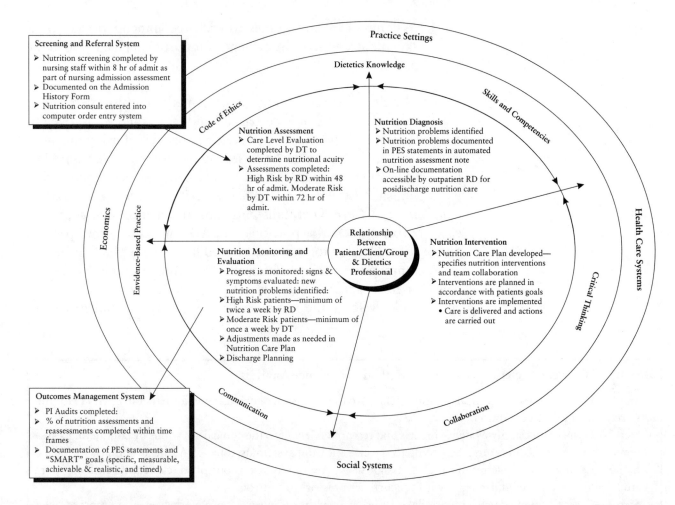

Figure 1.3 Example of Nutrition Care Process and Model in practice. Adapted from Lacey K, Pritchett E. Nutrition care process and model: ADA adopts road map to quality care and outcomes. *J Am Diet Assoc.* 2003;103:1061–1072, with permission from American Dietetic Association.

steps, developed through a consultative process by experts and practitioners, that incorporates current professional knowledge and available research and clearly defines the level, content, and frequency of nutrition care that is appropriate for a disease or condition in typical settings. In other words, the early protocols were consensus based and included references to support the recommendations they contained.

Since 2001, ADA and the Quality Management Committee have required adherence to more stringent development and revision processes to ensure that the protocols can be called *evidence based*. The more stringent process involves a stepwise progression:

1. Defining clinical questions to be answered
2. Identifying and analyzing literature that answers the clinical questions
3. Refining the original clinical questions into recommendations that are incorporated into the protocol

4. Assigning evidence grades to each recommendation to indicate the strength of the evidence supporting its inclusion in the protocol

Box 1.5 describes the evidence analysis method in more detail (37). The designation "Evidence-Based Guide for Practice" is given to an MNT Protocol that has been developed or revised using the more stringent process. The Evidence-Based Guides are available from ADA only in CD-ROM format, and they replace any earlier versions that were published by ADA in *Medical Nutrition Therapy Across the Continuum of Care*. Dietitians and clinical nutrition managers can check the product catalog portion of the ADA Web site or the Products and Services Catalog for new and revised Evidence-Based Guides.

A common format is used for all MNT Guides and MNT Protocols. The first page, the Summary Page, provides an overview of the entire guide. Refer to the Summary Page of the Type 2 diabetes melli-

---

Box 1.5   American Dietetic Association's Method of Evidence Analysis

- **Step 1—Formulate a set of clinical questions** related to the provision of medical nutrition therapy (MNT) for the selected diagnosis or condition.
- **Step 2—Gather and classify evidence reports and research** relevant to the clinical questions by conducting a systematic search of the literature. According to the classification system used by ADA, the level on the evidence hierarchy is noted by the letter of the class assigned; eg, A = randomized controlled (clinical) trial; B = cohort study; and C = nonrandomized trial with concurrent or historical controls.
- **Step 3—Critically appraise each report.** Each report or article is summarized on a worksheet, and a score is given based on the evidence quality and its relevance to the clinical questions. One of three scores is assigned: a plus sign (+) indicates a report that clearly addresses the issues of inclusion/exclusion, bias, generalizability, and data collection and analysis; a minus sign (–) indicates a report that does not clearly address these issues; a zero (0) indicates a report that is neither exceptionally strong nor exceptionally weak.
- **Step 4—Summarize the evidence in a conclusion statement.** The original clinical questions are answered by stating them as recommendations, known as *conclusion statements,* that can be incorporated into the Evidence-Based Guide.
- **Step 5—Grade the strength of evidence supporting the conclusion statement.** A grade indicates the overall strength or weakness of the evidence related to the clinical question and the recommendations being made. One of four grades is assigned: Grade I = good evidence with results from studies of strong design to answer the clinical question; Grade II = fair evidence (ie, the results are from studies of strong design, but there is uncertainty about the conclusion because of inconsistencies among results or design inconsistencies, or the results are from studies of weaker design but the results have been confirmed in separate studies); Grade III = the results are from a limited number of studies of weak design for answering the clinical question; or Grade IV = based on the recommendations of experts in the area based on their clinical experience but lacking support from research studies.
- **Step 6—Apply the research to practice by implementing the MNT Evidence-Based Guide and its recommendations.**
- **Step 7—Evaluate aggregate outcomes data, and review and update the guide based on these results,** along with new research that has become available since guide development. ADA has established a 2- to 3-year revision cycle for all MNT Evidence-Based Guides and MNT Protocols.

Source: Adapted with permission from American Dietetic Association Scientific Affairs and Research. *ADA Evidence Analysis Guide.* 2nd ed. Chicago, Ill: American Dietetic Association; 2003.

tus MNT Guide (see Figure 1.2). Other parts of each guide are the Flow Sheet, Session Process, Progress Note, and Bibliography. Each guide lists the setting in which it is to be used at the top of the Summary Page. Generally, guides are intended for use in outpatient care, ambulatory care, and private practice settings, although a few are appropriate for use in home care and long-term care settings. The Summary Page also lists the number of MNT interventions, the length of each intervention, suggested intervals between interventions, and suggested content of MNT for each session. The information on MNT sessions provides valuable guidance in estimating time requirements for MNT interventions.

ADA Position Statements and Papers

ADA has published position papers on a variety of topics that serve as a resource to dietitians and dietetic technicians about appropriate nutrition intervention for disease prevention and treatment. The position papers also can be used to determine the appropriateness of existing staff roles. More important, the content of some papers provides direction for new and expanded roles that can increase the visibility of dietetics professionals.

Position papers cover a wide range of topics, such as nutrition and lifestyle for a healthy pregnancy outcome, oral health and nutrition, cost-effectiveness of MNT, and nutrition services in managed care. A list of the current position papers by category was published in the February 2003 *Journal of the American Dietetic Association*. (38) Position papers can be accessed on the ADA Web site (*http://www.eatright.org/positions.html*) (39). Although high standards always have accompanied the development of position papers, this development must now adhere to the same evidence-based process that is required for developing the ADA Evidence-Based Guides.

A wide variety of factors must be considered in assessing staffing needs. Five important areas have been identified and described in detail:

1. The facility's mission, vision, populations served, and operations
2. Department services and operations, focusing on clinical nutrition services and the competencies and skill mix needed by staff
3. Legislation related to required patient care activities and the scope of practice of clinical nutrition staff
4. Accreditation standards to identify requirements that affect staffing, patient care, and assessment of performance
5. Professional practice issues and guidelines for patient care for specific patient populations

A regular assessment of these factors is needed to incorporate changes that occur over time and ensure continued relevance of the plan in meeting facility and department needs, regulations, standards,

ASSESSING STAFF NEEDS SUMMARY

and professional accountabilities. Once these factors have been evaluated, a staffing plan can be developed.

REFERENCES

1. Agency for Healthcare Quality and Research. Fact sheet: databases and related resources from HCUP. Available at: *http://www.ahcpr.gov/data/hcup/datahcup.htm*. Accessed October 12, 2003.

2. *2003 Hospital Accreditation Standards: Tools for Performance Measurement in Health Care: A Quick Reference Guide.* Oakbrook Terrace, Ill: Joint Commission Resources; 2002.

3. *American Dietetic Association Medical Nutrition Therapy Evidence-Based Guides for Practice* [CD-ROMs]. Chicago, Ill: American Dietetic Association; 2001.

4. Silverman MR, Gregoire MB, Lafferty LJ, Dowling RA. Current and future practices in hospital foodservice. *J Am Diet Assoc.* 2000;100:76–80.

5. Kwon J, Gilmore SA, Oakland MJ, Shelley MC II. Clinical dietetics changes due to cost-reduction activities in health care systems. *J Am Diet Assoc.* 2001; 101:1347–1350.

6. Performance, Proficiency, and Value Tactical Workgroup of the American Dietetic Association House of Delegates. Performance, proficiency, and value of the dietetics professional. *J Am Diet Assoc.* 2002;102:1304–1315.

7. Bryk JA, Soto TK. Report on the 1999 Membership Database of the American Dietetic Association. *J Am Diet Assoc.* 2001;101:947–953.

8. Salary Survey Work Group of the American Dietetic Association. Report on the ADA 2002 Dietetics Compensation and Benefits Survey. *J Am Diet Assoc.* 2003;103:243–255.

9. *Pediatric Nutrition Care Level Evaluation Process.* Nashville, Tenn: Vanderbilt University Medical Center; 2004.

10. Commission on Accreditation for Dietetics Education. Foundation knowledge and skills and competency requirements for entry-level dietetic technicians. Available at: *http://www.eatright.com/cade/standards.html*. Accessed May 13, 2003.

11. Ebiasah RP, Schneider PJ, Pedersen CA. Survey to evaluate certification in nutrition support pharmacy practice. *JPEN J Parenter Enteral Nutr.* 2002;26: 165–173.

12. Schneider PJ. Crossing the quality chasm: building a safe nutrition system. *JPEN J Parenter Enteral Nutr.* 2002;26:219–225.

13. Agency for Healthcare Research and Quality. Nutritional support. Chap. 33 in Making health care safer: a critical analysis of patient safety practices. Available at: *http://www.ahcpr.gov/clinic/ptsafety*. Accessed October 13, 2003.

14. Commission on Dietetic Registration. Laws that regulate dietitians/nutritionists. Available at: *http://www.cdrnet.org/certiciations/licensure/index.htm*. Accessed October 11, 2003.

15. Lacey K, Pritchett E. Nutrition Care Process and Model: ADA adopts road map to quality care and outcomes management. *J Am Diet Assoc.* 2003;103: 1061–1072.

16. Medicare program; revisions to payment policies and five-year review of and adjustments to the relative values units under the physician fee schedule for calendar year 2002: final rule. 66 *Federal Register* 55275–55281 (2001) (codified at 42 CFR 405).

17. Program Memorandum Intermediaries. Medical nutrition therapy (MNT) services for beneficiaries with diabetes or renal disease—policy change. Transmittal A-02–115. November 1, 2002. Available at: http://cms.hhs.gov/manuals/pm_trans/A02115.pdf. Accessed October 12, 2003.

18. American Dietetic Association. Medicare MNT Benefits and Resources. Available at: *http://www.eatright.org/Member/PolicyInitiatives/83_8722.cfm*. Accessed October 12, 2003.

19. *2004 Hospital Accreditation Standards (HAS)*. Chicago, Ill: Joint Commission on Accreditation of Healthcare Organizations; 2004.

20. Hiller L, Lowery JC, Davis JA, Shore CJ, Striplin DT. Nutritional status classification in the Department of Veterans Affairs. *J Am Diet Assoc.* 2001;101: 786–792.

21. VA Health Services Research and Development. Center for Practice Management and Outcomes Research. VA clinical nutrition staffing model. 1999. Available at: http://*www.hsrd.ann-arbor.med.va.gov/clinutstaf_jcl.htm*. Accessed May 13, 2003.

22. *Hospital Patient Assessment: Meeting the Challenges*. Chicago, Ill: Joint Commission on Accreditation of Healthcare Organizations; 2003.

23. Joint Commission on Accreditation of Healthcare Organizations. Frequently asked questions about staffing effectiveness. Available at: *http://www.jcaho. org/ accredited+organizations/hospitals/standards/hospital+faqs/manage+human+res/ planning/staffing+effectiveness.htm*. Accessed May 13, 2003.

24. American Dietetic Association and the Commission on Dietetic Registration. Code of Ethics for the Profession of Dietetics. *J Am Diet Assoc.* 1999;99: 109–113.

25. American Dietetic Association. Code of Ethics for the Profession of Dietetics. Available at: http://www.eatright.org/Member/Governance/index_18917.cfm. Accessed October 11, 2003.

26. Standards of Practice Task Force. The American Dietetic Association Standards of Professional Practice for Dietetics Professionals. *J Am Diet Assoc.* 1998; 98:83–87.

27. American Dietetic Association. Standards of Professional Practice. Available at: *http://www.eatright.org/Member/83_9468.cfm*. Accessed February 6, 2004.

28. Diabetes Care and Education Dietetic Practice Group. Scope of practice for qualified dietetics professionals in diabetes care and education. *J Am Diet Assoc.* 2000;100:1205–1207.

29. American Dietetic Association and American Society for Parenteral and Enteral Nutrition. Standards of Practice for the Nutrition Support Dietitian. Available at: *www.nutritioncare.org/profdev/rdstandards.pdf*. Accessed October 12, 2003.

30. Dietetic Practice Audit Panels of 1997–98, 1998–99, and 1999–2000 of the Commission on Dietetic Registration. 2000 Commission on Dietetic Registration dietetics practice audit. *J Am Diet Assoc.* 2002;102:270–292.

31. Inman-Felton A, Rops MS. *Ensuring Staff Competence: A Guide for Meeting JCAHO Competence Standards in All Settings*. Chicago, Ill: American Dietetic Association; 1998.

32. Moore C. In pursuit of competitive market advantage: compensation for clinical nutrition skills. *Future Dimensions Clin Nutr Manage.* 2003;22(1):1–7.

33. *Job Descriptions: Models for the Dietetics Profession*. Chicago, Ill: American Dietetic Association; 2003.

34. American Dietetic Association and Morrison Health Care. *Medical Nutrition Therapy Across the Continuum of Care.* Chicago, Ill: American Dietetic Association; 1996.

35. American Dietetic Association and Morrison Health Care. *Medical Nutrition Therapy Across the Continuum of Care.* Suppl 1. Chicago, Ill: American Dietetic Association; 1997.

36. American Dietetic Association and Morrison Health Care. *Medical Nutrition Therapy Across the Continuum of Care.* 2nd ed. Chicago, Ill: American Dietetic Association; 1998.

37. American Dietetic Association Scientific Affairs and Research. *ADA Evidence Analysis Guide.* 2nd ed. Chicago, Ill: American Dietetic Association; 2003.

38. Position paper update. *J Am Diet Assoc.* 2003;103:241–242.

39. American Dietetic Association. Position Paper Index. Available at: http://www.eatright.org/Member/PolicyInitiatives/8474_17299.cfm. Accessed October 11, 2003.

CHAPTER 2

Identifying New Opportunities

Chapter 1 describes how to assess current needs for clinical nutrition staffing. It briefly mentions assessing needs for new programs and services in this process. However, the topics of program development and expansion deserve more in-depth consideration because of the pivotal role they play in the evolution of dietetic practice. To ensure that the dietetics profession is at the forefront in health promotion and disease prevention and treatment, managers and clinical nutrition staff must be assertive in creating demand for nutrition programs and services, expanding practice roles to accommodate actual and potential needs, and establishing partnerships and collaborations within the health care environment to support the implementation of the programs and services. The present chapter provides background information on opportunities for creating new programs and services and for expanding existing ones. Areas for innovation and expansion are discussed, and examples are provided.

OPPORTUNITIES FOR PROGRAM DEVELOPMENT AND EXPANSION

Organizational Changes

Health care facilities are not static institutions. Like other areas of the culture and economy, they are affected by many factors that produce what at times seems like constant change. Areas of change that affect facilities and their priorities include the following:

- National, state, and local economies
- National and state legislation
- Accreditation standards
- Contracts with, and reimbursement from, payers
- Cost of providing care
- Advances in technology
- Populations served, including demographic changes in the communities served
- Health promotion and disease prevention and treatment priorities, both national and local
- Ability to recruit qualified staff and retain existing workforce

A periodic reassessment of staffing needs and of the adequacy of the staffing plan is needed to incorporate and plan for anticipated and actual changes.

Reimbursement for Nutrition Services and Medical Nutrition Therapy

Because of variation in payer policies for reimbursement of medical nutrition therapy (MNT) and the ongoing changes in health care and reimbursement policies, it is not surprising that managers and clinical nutrition staff find it difficult to understand and keep up with policies that affect their own reimbursement practices. However, because coverage and payment for programs and services determine financial viability, ongoing attention to reimbursement issues is warranted.

The American Dietetic Association (ADA) is committed to assisting its members in these efforts and to advocating for continued and expanded coverage of nutrition services by third party payers. To accomplish these goals, staff on the Quality, Outcomes, and Coverage Team have implemented a multipronged initiative designed to maintain oversight of legislative and financing processes affecting coverage of nutrition programs and services. At each opportunity, staff advocate for both coverage and procedures that support coverage (eg, the approval by the American Medical Association of *Current Procedural Terminology* [CPT] codes for MNT). In addition, many affiliates and dietetic practice groups (DPGs) have established volunteer positions within their organizations that are charged with providing members with reimbursement updates and assistance in obtaining payment for services at the local level. Readers can access the ADA report on legislative and policy initiatives at http://*www.eatright.com/images/leadership/nptf.pdf* (1).

An article in the February 2002 *Journal of the American Dietetic Association* provided a scan of the reimbursement environment for nutrition programs and services (2). The authors presented issues surrounding payment for health care in general and summarized descriptive data from interviews with a variety of key decision makers in health care firms and managed care organizations. They also compared the information from these interviews, which were conducted in 2002, with information obtained during a series of similar interviews 3 years earlier.

The authors noted that fundamental changes in coverage and reimbursement strategies are taking place in response to both the rising costs of providing health care and consumer demands for services. They found that coverage decisions are being made at many levels, including the consumer level. Consumers are demanding more input into decisions, in part because of having to shoulder increased out-of-pocket expenses for their health care.

Interview feedback indicated changes in perception of the importance of nutrition care and MNT by the key decision makers, along with increased MNT coverage and reimbursement. At the time of the

---

Strategies to Increase Reimbursement

Registered dietitans (RDs) and RD managers can be proactive in their approach to seeking increased reimbursement by doing the following:

- Contacting plan case managers to request additional MNT sessions when patients are making progress toward goals.
- Collecting and summarizing outcomes for thier patient populations (ie, patients with the same diagnosis or condition or patients having the same procedure).
- Sharing outcome data with physicians to increase referrals ind build support for reimbursement.
- Informing plan benefits coordinators about the *ADA Medical Nutrition Therapy Evidence-Based Guides for Prctice* and sharing outcome data to define coverage requirements and demonstrate the impact of coverage, especially vcoverage for more than one MNT session.
- Informing contract managers and plan decision makers about the *ADA Medical Ntrition Therapy Evidence-Bases Guides for Practice* and sharing outcome data resulting from their use with patients.
- Reporting successes to colleagues and mentoring them in their own efforts to seek increased reimbursement.

second set of interviews, most plans directly covered MNT, in contrast to the limited direct coverage that was noted at the time of the first interviews. The geographic differences in coverage noted during the first interviews had declined in the 3-year interval as well.

Opportunities for dietetics professionals were identified. Because of increased decision making by consumers, dietetics professionals were encouraged to differentiate their services from similar services provided by individuals with lesser qualifications. The authors noted that consumers were often not aware of the added value of programs and services provided by dietetics professionals. They recommended that outcomes data be used to market programs and services to consumers and payers, and that customer service and satisfaction be a major focus.

The report noted that new and integrated models for care and disease management are being implemented for chronic disease and weight management. Clinical nutrition staff must understand the new models, their multiple streams of patient referral, and the procedures used to identify and stratify health and disease risk. They also must understand how to identify and implement nutrition interventions for patients at the different levels of risk. Opportunities exist for registered dietitians (RDs) to be leaders of interdisciplinary teams, case managers, and managers of disease management programs.

Other Sources of Financial Support

Managers and clinical nutrition staff often enlist the support of the managers and staff of other departments for nutrition programs and services. Support can take many forms, including payment for all or part of the cost of the RD salary and benefits or other costs associated with the program. For example, the marketing department of a facility or health system may have funds to cover the costs of marketing a nutrition program or service to the community. Collaborations must be built and positive working relationships established well in advance of actual need for this type of support. Alternative sources of revenue, such as grants and foundation monies, also should be investigated.

When developing new programs and services and evaluating existing ones, it is essential that managers and clinical nutrition staff determine all costs for delivering the programs or services. They must consider direct and indirect expenses, as well as overhead expenses (eg, the costs of doing business, such as rent, telephone, and administrative support). Program approval and viability usually depend on generating sufficient revenues to cover or exceed costs, through charges to clients or the receipt of other revenue.

Population Health and Disease Management

Opportunities exist for RDs to be involved in population health and disease management programs. Population health programs offer a different, though complementary, approach to traditional health care.

They focus on groups of people instead of individual patients. The programs emphasize trends in society that can have either a positive or negative impact on national or regional health, the broad impact of good health or poor health on society, and the groups of people within our society who do not access traditional systems of health care. Population health programs also tend to emphasize environmental factors that affect health behaviors, such as income, education, employment, and housing conditions (3).

Responsibilities of RDs working in population-based health programs are broad and generally not limited to direct patient care. Table 2.1 summarizes the roles for RDs engaged in population health programs for people with diabetes mellitus, as described in an article by Faye Wong in the Spring 2003 issue of *On the Cutting Edge,* the newsletter of the Diabetes Care and Education DPG (4).

Case and Care Management

Dietitians are well suited for roles as case and care managers for patients with complex medical conditions, especially conditions that

Table 2.1   Registered Dietitians' Roles in Population Health

Role	Examples of Activities
Health communication	• Translating research and new data into health messages • Developing television and print advertisements • Testing messages and products on intended audiences
Education	• Developing curricula and training materials that can be used by community health workers • Educating administrators, legislators, and community health officials
Coalition building	• Initiating and implementing collaborations to work together to address health issues
• Statewide and community assessment	• Reviewing demographic and health data to characterize rates of diseases and risk factors • Designing new data collection efforts through surveys and surveillance systems
• Improving systems of care	• Developing and implementing standards of care • Developing systems to monitor compliance and report performance • Identifying and implementing strategies to improve performance
• Direct care	• Providing one-to-one and group interventions to clients of community health centers, primary health care clinics, minority health clinics, and health department clinics

Source: Data are from reference 4.

have a strong link with MNT. Patients with complex conditions must access complicated and often fragmented health care systems, and they must obtain costly services and products for treatment. RD case managers can facilitate access to these needed services and products. They can monitor outcomes and adjust treatments or facilitate adjustments, and they can coordinate communication among multiple layers of health care providers. Examples of diseases and conditions ideal for RD case management are diabetes mellitus, obesity, and inborn errors of metabolism, such as phenylketonuria.

In recent years, home health care companies have experienced serious reductions in funding and payment for services, added requirements for data collection to comply with new regulations, and increased patient acuity. As a result, some agencies have closed or consolidated.

Even before these changes in the home care arena, RDs were not widely employed by home care agencies. Schiller and colleagues surveyed home care administrators in 1998 and found that more than 50% of the administrators surveyed did not employ a consultant dietitian. Survey respondents attributed this situation to the lack of both third party reimbursement and physician requests for RD services (5).

The nutrition care of patients on home nutrition support needs to be coordinated, an ideal role for RD case managers. Hospital-based RDs, especially certified nutrition support dietitians (CNSDs), are well positioned to fill this role. In addition to providing inpatient MNT, they can establish links between inpatient and home nutrition support and the providers in both settings. They can monitor patient progress in achieving nutrition goals through telephone communication and on-line accessing of laboratory reports. And they can communicate with members of the health care team across the care continuum, preventing problems when possible and identifying the problems that do occur early on. This early identification of problems can avert costly emergency room visits and readmissions to treat dehydration and problems with metabolic control.

The challenge for RDs working with home care patients is to develop high-quality, efficient systems of care and to ensure their own financial viability, whether they are based in hospitals or home care agencies. An article in the December 2002 issue of *Support Line,* the newsletter of the Dietitians in Nutrition Support (DNS) DPG, provided a model of care and tools for use by RDs interested in filling this niche (6).

Customized One-to-One MNT Counseling

Patient-centered approaches to nutrition counseling are advocated to promote the dietary changes and long-term adherence to interventions needed to produce desired health outcomes. Patient-centered counseling has a firm theoretical foundation in consumer information processing theory, the health belief model, the stages of change model, social cognitive theory, and behavioral self-management (7). MNT is tailored to clients' stages of change. Clients are active participants in the goal-setting process, and counseling focuses on identifying and resolving the challenges clients encounter in making and maintaining their changes.

Traditionally, training programs for RDs and dietetic technicians, registered (DTRs), have provided little opportunity to develop competency in patient-centered counseling. Limited training, coupled with a lack of opportunity to hone skills because of infrequent client follow-up, makes understandable the inexperience of many RDs with this approach to care. However, to be effective MNT counselors in the future, RDs must learn and use this set of skills. Fortunately, the ADA recognized this training need and incorporated skill building on motivational interviewing and patient-centered counseling strategies into the Commission on Dietetic Registration (CDR) Adult and Pediatric Weight Management Certificate workshops.

Work has been done toward the development of a tool, the Nutrition Quality of Life (NQOL) measure, that RDs can use to individualize MNT. The tool was developed using qualitative research methods, including interviews with focus groups of RDs and patients. It is intended to measure the impact of MNT interventions on clients' quality of life. General areas measured by the tool include physical, social, and psychological domains. Specific categories measured include readiness to change, food impact, self-image, and self-efficacy (8).

The client's NQOL is measured prior to initial and follow-up MNT sessions. At an initial session, the tool is used to establish a patient-specific baseline and provide the RD with insight into actual and potential adherence issues so that appropriate support can be provided from the beginning of the counseling process. The tool's use during follow-up sessions allows RDs and clients to assess clients' adaptation to the MNT interventions from the perspective of quality of life. MNT counseling can be targeted to address identified problems. The NQOL tool can be found at *http://www.bouve.neu.edu/nercoa.html* (9).

In addition to these expanded strategies for counseling clients, RDs now have access to new sources of information about dietary requirements and the upper limits of safe intake of nutrients in the Dietary Reference Intakes (10–14). They also have access to expanded lists of nutrient and bioactive components of foods and to laboratory results that focus on very individualized risk factors (eg, the type and size of clients' lipoprotein particles). Taken together, these sources of information provide RDs with the opportunity to customize their recommendations to clients on food and nutrient intake, patterns of food consumption, and use of dietary supplements in a way that cannot be matched by others seeking to give dietary advice.

The next horizon for RDs is nutritional genomics, an area of research and practice that evaluates the effect of dietary factors on the expression of different genes and the effect of genes on the utilization and metabolism of nutrients. Not only does nutritional genomics have the potential to transform the science of nutrition; it also has the potential to transform the provision of MNT. Predictions are for future practice that incorporates nutritional genomics and allows precise customization of MNT interventions, similar to the specificity now provided to patients with phenylketonuria (15). For example, it may be possible to counsel clients to reduce their risk of chronic disease based on an understanding of their genes, identification of early biomarkers for disease, and determination of the impact of gene expressions on nutrient metabolism.

An example cited by Janet King in her interview in the *Journal of the American Dietetic Association* underscores the importance of individualization of MNT recommendations (15). She described the research of Ronald Krauss, who has shown that a low-fat diet has a negative impact on the lipid profiles of some individuals, resulting in an increased risk of cardiovascular disease rather than the reduction in risk that might be expected. Apparently, people who have initially high levels of the small, dense lipoproteins that are associated with an increased risk of cardiovascular disease respond to a low-fat diet as expected—that is, with a reduction in the small, dense lipoproteins. However, the genetic response to a low-fat diet of approximately half of those individuals with initially high levels of large, low-density lipoproteins is an increase in their levels of small, dense lipoproteins, thus increasing their risk of cardiovascular disease (15). Although there is clearly much to learn about nutritional genomics, the door has been opened to a new and exciting era of MNT. RDs must build the skills today that will enable them to capitalize on the opportunities of the future.

Advances in Technology

Many RDs have expanded their use of technology in the past few years, and others are still learning to do so. RDs must be technologically savvy and knowledgeable about available technology, as current technology is rapidly replaced by ever-newer tools and programs. Expansion of the use of technology by restaurants and supermarkets will provide RDs with opportunities for consumer education and research.

The following are examples of ways to use current technology for different components of the nutrition care process:

- *Assessing nutritional requirements.* RDs can perform indirect calorimetry and use the results to predict clients' energy needs.
- *Assessing dietary intake.* Clients with digital cameras or cell phones with video capability can take and transmit photographs of their intake to the RD for review. Clients can use Web-based tools and programs to analyze and track their intake, plan their menus, and communicate their results to the RD prior to

their appointment time. This process saves RD and client time and reinforces the importance of self-monitoring. The December 2002 *Journal of the American Dietetic Association* includes an article that summarizes the capabilities of available tools and programs to assess dietary intake, including several free programs that offer many options to clients and are user-friendly (16).

- *Providing on-line client education, counseling, and communication.* RDs can use Web sites to offer their services and can facilitate chat rooms. They can participate in videoconferences with patients in outlying sites to minimize travel and allow limited physical assessment.

Trends Affecting Dietetics

As part of its work to define a new strategic plan, ADA conducted an environmental scan. In completing the scan, ADA identified more than 100 issues, trends, and events that are likely to affect the organization and its members in the next decade. The information from this process was given to a consultant group, Leading Futurists, LLC, in Washington, DC. The consultants sorted, validated, and organized the trends into a report for the ADA Board of Directors that was published in the *Journal of the American Dietetic Association* (17). The report provided insight into potential changes needed in the delivery of existing nutrition services and programs, and it identified opportunities to meet needs that are anticipated to arise in the next decade. A sample of trends described in the summary, along with their potential impact, is listed in Table 2.2 (17). Another resource on trends is the book *Bowling Alone,* by Robert Putnam (18).

Strategic Plan

In January 2003, the ADA Board of Directors approved the 2004–2008 strategic plan. Included in the plan are a new mission and vision statement, five priority areas for nutrition and dietetics, and new strategic goals (19). Although intended to provide direction to initiatives of the ADA, the DPGs, and affiliates, the priority areas also provide insight into the patient populations and types of programs likely to be needed at the community and facility levels.

LEADER VISIONS Leaders within the ADA provide information and insight that managers and clinical nutrition staff can use in redefining their roles and in developing and planning programs and services for the future of dietetics. There are many ways to access and share ideas with ADA leaders: during interactions at national, state, and local meetings; by reading articles and books the leaders have authored; and through e-mail correspondence and participation on Listservs. The ADA has

Table 2.2   **Key Trends Affecting Dietetics**

Category	Trends	Potential Opportunities
Changes in the population	• US population is aging. • Average lifespan will be prolonged. • By 2010, 120 million Americans, or 40% of the population, will be diagnosed with a chronic condition or disease.	Programs in diverse settings: • Ambulatory care • Home care • Community-based care
Changing values and attitudes	• Americans continue to emphasize the issues and needs of children and the elderly. • Concerns about time shape daily life as people face time pressures inherent in society.	Programs for subsets of the population: • Pediatrics • Seniors Services that save time: • On-line and telephonic nutrition counseling and education
Challenges of the modern lifestyle	• More Americans have sedentary lifestyles. • More workers have computer-related occupations. • Children and teenagers are spending more time in front of the TV, video screen, or computer screen.	Participation in broad coalitions: • School programs • Community-based initiatives Integrated weight management and exercise programs
Work life and the workforce	• American families are collectively spending more time at work. • More workers telecommute some or all of the time.	Nutrition programs and services based in the workplace World Wide Web–based services for telecommuters
Technology-driven lifestyle changes and new issues	• Genetics and biotechnology are driving new technologies and issues.	Counseling services designed to help people understand the emerging relationships among genetics, biotechnology, nutrition, the environment, and health
Health care shortfalls at a time when preventive care is being advocated	• More Americans go without health insurance some or all of the time. • Wide disparities in access to health care continue. • Obesity is a growing public issue. • Diabetes mellitus is an emerging concern as its incidence increases.	Programs for emerging disease populations: • Pediatric type 2 diabetes • "Prediabetes" • Pediatric weight management Programs for underserved populations

Source: Data are from reference 17.

been fortunate to have a wealth of visionary leaders and a large pool of members from which new leaders are emerging. This section shares the insights and visions of three ADA leaders.

Past ADA president Sara Parks, PhD, MBA, RD, presented the 2001 Lenna Frances Cooper Memorial Lecture on October 23, 2001, at the ADA Food and Nutrition Conference and Exhibition. In her presentation, "The Fractured Ant Hill: A New Architecture for Sustaining the Future," she stressed that members must embrace the reality that consumers have changed. They are, and will continue to be, better educated, increasingly adept at the use of technology, and in possession of more disposable income. According to Parks, consumers have partially rejected the standardization and efficiencies of health care systems, as evidenced by their turning to alternative therapies and self-care. They want personal attention to their needs and want to be addressed on their own terms—for example, getting information in small chunks and in a format they choose. Consumers also want to schedule MNT sessions according to their availability, not that of their RD providers. Parks also suggested that practitioners of the future become comfortable with reinventing practice roles numerous times during their careers and with the necessity for ongoing skill development. The lecture was published in its entirety in the January 2002 issue of the *Journal of the American Dietetic Association* (20).

In her October 2002 President's editorial, Julie O'Sullivan Maillet, PhD, RD, FADA, described her vision for dietetics professionals working in clinical settings in 2017, the year of the ADA's 100th anniversary (21). O'Sullivan Maillet envisioned that future clinical dietitians working in the outpatient setting will be nutrition therapists whose duties include the following:

- *Client assessment.* This assessment will be supported by on-line access to detailed health histories, data from body composition analyses, and serial diet histories.
- *Counseling.* Counseling will be (1) focused on determination of individual needs that are based on clients' age, genetics, body composition, health status, and lifestyle; (2) built on clients' awareness of the importance of healthy eating and the improved understanding of the roles of numerous phytochemicals; and (3) provided on-line and by telephone, as well as in person.
- *Partnering with patients.* This partnering will be exemplified by clients completing their own assessments of their progress.
- *Routine monitoring, assessment, and documentation of the outcomes of MNT.*

O'Sullivan Maillet envisioned that dietitians working in the inpatient setting will function in roles similar to those of today's nurse practitioners and advanced-practice nurses. They will write diet orders and participate in all feeding decisions, using care protocols and relying on their clinical expertise. They will be part of all health care teams and will use technology to record, document, and store food and nutrient intake; for example, photographs of patient trays before and after meals may be stored in computer databases.

In the 2002 Lenna Frances Cooper Memorial Lecture, presented at the October 2002 Food and Nutrition Conference and Exhibition, Marian Franz, MS, RD, CDE, described the impact that RDs have had on the management of diabetes mellitus. She noted that in people with type 2 diabetes mellitus, successful MNT produces a comparable reduction in the blood levels of hemoglobin A1C, which are used to assess blood glucose control over time, as oral hypoglycemia agents. This is a reduction of 2 percentage points in newly diagnosed individuals and 1 percentage point in people who have had diabetes for 4 years or more (22).

Franz emphasized that to have this positive impact, RDs must rely on the use of evidence-based interventions, routinely monitor the outcomes of MNT and self-management training, and manage the disease by ensuring that individual patient outcomes data serve as the basis for adjustments in treatment and education. (Box 2.1 provides an example of MNT disease management by an RD.) Franz concluded her presentation by outlining a vision for a future practice role: the advanced dietitian practitioner, whom she envisions having advanced education and treatment-ordering privileges, similar to the advanced nurse practitioner.

At first consideration, the visions of O'Sullivan Maillet and of Franz, which involve RDs with order-writing privileges, may seem out of reach to dietitians. However, RDs in some health systems already have order-writing privileges, also referred to as *clinical privileges*. Clinical privileges are defined as the ability to make specific, independent judgments determined to be appropriate for an individual health care provider such as an RD. They extend beyond merely taking verbal orders from physicians (23).

Box 2.1   Example of Medical Nutrition Therapy (MNT) Disease Management by a Registered Dietitian (RD)

At the client's 6-week MNT appointment, the RD reviews the laboratory data and determines whether or not the client's hemoglobin A1C level is below 7.5%.

If yes:

- MNT interventions are continued. The client's nutrition care plan is adjusted as needed to meet his health goals.
- The RD collaborates with the physician, as appropriate, regarding the possible need for reduction in oral hypoglycemic medication.

If no:

- The RD assesses the client's understanding of the MNT interventions, his ability to make changes in his diet and eating behaviors, the barriers and challenges he may encounter in trying to do so, and his willingness to make changes.
- When the client is willing to make changes, the RD renegotiates goals and establishes strategies with the client to achieve the goals.

If the client is unable to make changes, unwilling to do so, or both, the RD collaborates with the physician about the status of MNT goals and the possible need for medications to control diabetes mellitus.

The January 2002 *Journal of the American Dietetic Association* contained two articles on the topic of clinical privileges for RDs affiliated with health care systems. One article provided background information on the topic and a case example of implementation of clinical privileges by RDs in the military (24).

The second article described how RDs in a health system in Arizona used the performance improvement process to identify a patient safety issue and how they used this issue as the springboard for implementation of clinical privileges. Performance improvement data revealed that an excessive amount of time elapsed between documentation of RD recommendations for nutrition care and physicians' writing of orders for these recommendations. The RDs and their managers collaborated with the physicians and built acceptance for their proposal for clinical privileges, leading to its successful implementation (25). As discussed in Chapter 1, clinical privileges for staff with demonstrated competencies can be a key component of a career ladder.

The following pages explore the vision for future RD practice roles in the clinical setting through interviews with four ADA leaders: Susan Laramee, MS, RD, FADA, CNSD; Sylvia Escott-Stump, MA, RD; Elvira Q. Johnson, MS, RD, CDE; and Pamela Charney, MS, RD, CNSD.

In an interview with Mary Jo Kurko Coyne, MPH, RD, director for nutrition development at ARAMARK Healthcare Support Services, Kurko Coyne describes an initiative that she has spearheaded with her accounts to streamline inpatient nutrition education, shift RD resources to the outpatient setting, and initiate or expand MNT services in the outpatient setting.

Also included is an interview with Eve Callahan, RD, CNSD. Callahan was a bone marrow transplant (MBT) dietitian at Vanderbilt University Medical Center (VUMC) in Nashville, Tennessee, and a highly valued member of the BMT team during her tenure on it. The final interview is with Ellen Ladage, MS, RD, CNSD, a surgery dietitian at VUMC and care coordinator for patients on enteral nutrition support.

All interviews were conducted by the author, Christina Biesemeier. The interviewees are expressing their personal views and are not speaking on behalf of the American Dietetic Association.

INSIGHTS FROM THE EXPERTS: INTERVIEWS AND ESSAYS

Vision for the Future: An Interview With Susan Laramee, MS, RD, FADA, CNSD

Question: Describe your vision for the roles of the clinical dietitian in the year 2017, ADA's 100th anniversary. Inpatient setting?

SUSAN LARAMEE: RDs and DTRs will function in a very electronic way, using handheld devices (the next generation of PDAs [personal digital assistants], laptops, and WiFi [wireless computer network] technology) to complete all tasks. They will enter notes into their devices. The notes will be transmitted to servers for insertion into the medical record. They will use their devices to recall patient information. This will likely occur is some settings well before 2017, but the technology will be fully mature by that date. There will be no "diet office." All patient menu choices will be made using the "room service" model. Patients will demand control over their meal selections and will be able to make selections electronically from the bedside when they want to eat. Much of the tedious detail that we have built into patient service systems will go away.

RDs will become more politically savvy (This is essential for survival!) and will move out of the silos that are common in today's health care environment. They will become more aligned with the medical care team and more focused on how they can use their services to enhance the care of patients and achieve patient outcomes. They will look for ways to tailor nutrition services to meet the goals of the inpatient setting, rather than trying to "shoe horn" old models into changing systems. Enteral formulas will be customized for specific diseases.

Question: Outpatient setting?

SL: Increased focus will be placed on diets designed to prevent the impact of aging. There will be reimbursement for the management of chronic disease. Preventive care, which will be in high demand, will be self-pay. This will be an acceptable way of getting services for many, but will create a two-tier system of health care in our society—something that will likely become acceptable.

Patients will often bypass counseling for information on-line. Technology will permit patients needing nutrition counseling to have their sessions at home via computer and video hookups. Again, RDs will rely heavily on technology to provide services. Education materials will be customized for each patient, and preprinted materials will give way to customized materials.

Services will be offered under the "disease management" umbrella. RDs will increasingly manage these programs, supervising nurses and other allied health professionals. At the same time, RDs will less frequently have other RDs as their supervisors. RDs will move into counseling on physical activity and will gain expertise in developing exercise prescriptions. Diet and exercise will need to be aligned, and the advice will need to come from the same practitioner.

In all practice settings, there will be greater diversity among the membership of ADA, another "essential" for our rapidly changing world.

Question: How do these roles differ from current roles?

SL: There will much greater adoption and utilization of technology to eliminate activities that do not have meaningful outcomes. Inefficiencies will continue to be eliminated, and in some cases, services will be eliminated. Innovation will be rewarded, and the dietetic practitioner who is able to function solo in the workplace—that is, without an RD supervisor or dietetics network—will be most successful. The professional association will have greater value because it will be the network, education, and technological support that the increasing number of solo practitioners need.

Question: What needs to happen to make your vision a reality?

SL: RDs need to think differently. They need to learn more about the business side of food, health care, and nutrition and about how they can fit more effectively into their organizations. At the present time, they work with too much of an isolationist approach and, as a result, suffer the economic consequences, especially in their salaries. Clinical training needs to focus as much on developing the skills needed for managing in the work environment as it does on learning the clinical skills. By this I am referring to the need for these competencies:

- Forming alliances with others
- Working effectively on teams
- Leading others
- Presenting programs
- Developing plans and ideas in a way that motivates others to "buy their products"
- Advocating effectively with other providers for nutrition services
- Defining expectations of organizational leaders, and developing plans and tailoring services to meet these expectations

Scope of practice may need to be expanded to include the ability to make exercise recommendations. Remember that personal trainers do not hesitate to make suggestions on nutrition! Training will also need to include some of the skill sets for developing effective exercise plans for clients.

Vision for the Future: An Interview With Sylvia Escott-Stump, MA, RD

Question: Describe your vision for the roles of the clinical dietitian in the year 2017, ADA's 100th anniversary. Inpatient setting?

SYLVIA ESCOTT-STUMP: The clinical dietitian of 2017 will work in his or her own office suite in the hospital or nursing home setting. The clinical dietitian will also be in charge of the nutrition support teams, with a team for every 100 patients. This nutrition support team will include the RD leader, several DTRs, clerical assistance, and consultants from the medical and pharmacy departments. The RD will conduct in-depth assessments and will write orders for the medical record, to be implemented by various non—nutrition team members (RN, MD, RPh, speech therapist, etc). Charting is electronic and confidential. RD positions will require a master's degree in medical nutrition therapy or nutritional science; RDs will hold certification as "medical nutritionists." The positions will be exciting, challenging and extremely rewarding—no more "I can't believe we are not recognized."

Question: Outpatient setting?

SE: In 2017, some outpatient dietitians will work as *partners* in practices with family practitioners, internists, pediatricians, OB-GYN specialists, gastroenterologists, and endocrinologists. Other outpatient dietitians of 2017 will work in their own office suites, next door to health care facilities such as hospitals and long-term care facilities. Each office will be arranged to allow one-to-one counseling, prescheduled as needed according to patients' treatment plans. Patients will be brought to this area as they are now taken to physical therapy suites that are associated with health care facilities. The staff in the office suite will include several DTRs and clerical assistants. The RD will provide in-depth consultation and counseling to clients, and he or she will send a full report to the appropriate medical office for inclusion in all medical records. Charting will be electronic and confidential. RDs will be required to have a master's degree in a counseling or psychology field; they will hold certification as "nutrition therapists."

Question: How do these roles differ from current roles?

SE: They have increased recognition from peer health providers that reflect RDs' equal "status" and the levels of recognition accorded by peers for the work performed and the contributions to changes in health outcomes.

Question: What needs to happen to make your vision a reality?

SE: There needs to be stronger preparation at the master's degree level for RD clinicians. Perhaps we need to make the DTR the entry-level position for our profession (4-year degree), with the RD requiring a master's degree. I would also make the DTR the entry point for management dietitians and have the RD acquire an MBA or equivalent in hospitality management or a related business/management degree.

Perhaps it is time to compete more effectively with our allied health peers, who have moved several practitioner slots up a notch to master's and doctoral practice.

Vision for the Future: An Interview With Elvira Q. Johnson, MS, RD, CDE

Question: Describe your vision for the roles of the clinical dietitian in the year 2017, ADA's 100th anniversary. Inpatient setting?

ELVIRA Q. JOHNSON: With severely reduced lengths of stay and fewer hospitalizations, there will be few inpatient RD positions beyond advanced-practice nutrition support.

Question: Outpatient setting?

EJ: The majority of clinical dietetics positions will be in outpatient settings, where many RDs will work in small group practices. In the outpatient setting, the trend will be toward nutrition therapy practitioners, advanced-level clinicians who have master's degrees and have completed nutrition residencies. Advanced-practice clinicians will be essential in caring for patients with chronic diseases such as diabetes and cardiovascular disease. They will work with great autonomy and will be able to achieve significant clinical improvements with minimum use of medications, a necessity due to the high costs of medications. Most patient interactions and interventions will occur via electronic tools.

Question: How do these roles differ from current roles?

EJ: The advanced practitioner role will require advanced-level training. Advanced practitioners will have significant autonomy and respect, and also greater accountability for outcomes. They will need enhanced behavioral skills, as well as comprehensive clinical assessment competencies. Performance evaluations and compensation will be determined by clinical outcomes and client satisfaction.

Question: What needs to happen to make your vision a reality?

EJ: Additional research and irrefutable evidence of the impact of clinical dietetics professionals on improved outcomes are essential. They will lead to enhanced reimbursement, compensation, and role definition redesign. Advanced educational and training programs will be needed to prepare RDs to be advanced practitioners.

Vision for the Future: An Interview With Pamela Charney, MS, RD, CNSD

Question: Describe your vision for the roles of the clinical dietitian in the year 2017, ADA's 100th anniversary. Inpatient setting?

PAMELA CHARNEY: I see the clinical dietitian as an indispensable member of the team, no longer the "phantom in the medical record." My vision also includes a much more flexible team structure with roles shifting according to patient needs, and smooth transition of duties between all members. We see this in some institutions now, where pharmacy, nursing, and dietetics all share management of nutrition support patients. More and more, physicians are being pulled in many different directions and need to rely on well-trained, assertive, intelligent partners to ensure that patient care is provided in a safe, cost-effective manner, and that we have the outcomes to support our actions. Once we have the data and the training to use those data, there will be no doubt in anyone's mind of the importance of the clinical dietitian!

I also see less and less patient education happening in the inpatient setting. Length of stay is shorter, reimbursement is not possible, and there is just so much happening during the inpatient stay that education will be only on those "survival skills" needed to go home. We will need to learn to shorten our message and include the sound bites that patients are used to from media, and prepare them to follow up as outpatients. This will include even nutrition support patients. Get them the skills they need to get to the outpatient/home care folks!

Question: Outpatient setting?

PC: There will be so many roles for outpatient dietitians! As we learn more about the human genome, we'll realize that there is no such thing as a diet for all. We'll learn to individualize even more, depending on genetic makeup. It will be important for ADA to capitalize on this, as there are so many others out there with less accurate information. The public is drawn to glitz, and we will need to learn how to operate in an increasingly techno-savvy world.

Question: How do these roles differ from current roles?

PC: I think that RDs today are often not vocal enough. When we do get vocal, we are seen as whining (which may very well be the case!). In order to increase staffing, we will have to show the impact of increased staff on patient outcomes. We will have to show that having that additional FTEs [full-time equivalents] leads to patients' going home sooner, or having fewer complications, or somehow saving money. I think the key now is going to be saving money, not spending more on labs or formulas or even more staff without showing how that cost leads to savings down the road.

We will need to learn business skills. I've seen other professions (nursing, pharmacy) become much more business oriented, and it's led to some new, expanded roles for them. We are often too nurturing for our own good. We have to learn to talk the language of our administrators.

Question: What needs to happen to make your vision a reality?

PC: Education and training are keys. I sometimes wonder if we need to look at where other professions are headed and evaluate our own training. Is a 4-year degree enough? Should internships be expanded? I remember when surgical residencies were 4 years; now they are in training for 5 to 6 years. We might need to accept the fact that the information can no longer be condensed. We also have to look at the preceptor system we currently have. Sometimes folks just don't make good preceptors; sometimes they just need to learn how to teach.

I also think we have to send our students and interns out to learn how to administer health care. Things are so complicated, and you often don't get a complete picture when you spend all your training in one area of a facility.

Innovations in Practice: An Interview With
Mary Jo Kurko Coyne, MPH, RD

ARAMARK Healthcare Support Services is implementing a comprehensive patient education initiative in our accounts that involves two phases and spans the care continuum from the inpatient to the outpatient setting. In phase one of this initiative, we have made the decision to focus inpatient education on survival skills, that is, the key messages that are intended to help patients avoid harm or get started on what will be an ongoing program of change in food choices and eating behaviors. Dietitians and dietetic technicians assist patients in selecting one step to take after discharge, until they can receive more information during outpatient follow-up.

We have revised all of our education materials to the sixth-grade reading level. Most materials list three bullet points—that is, the key messages—with a short explanation of each point. A few materials list up to five bullet points.

There will be exceptions to our "survival skills approach." Examples of exceptions are patients who are from out of town and unable to return for follow-up and older patients whose caregivers are present and interested in knowing more about nutrition interventions than just survival skills.

We anticipate several positive results from this first phase of our initiative. First, patients will have a better understanding of the actions they need to take in the initial days and weeks after their discharge from the hospital. We know that patients are often overwhelmed by multiple discharge instructions. By keeping our nutrition message simple, we increase the likelihood that it will be understood and used. Second, staff satisfaction will be increased, because their focus is on a few essential points of information, not the many details that can be provided when patients are feeling better and able to participate in interactive learning. Third, we anticipate that the RD time saved by streamlining inpatient education can be reallocated to the outpatient setting, providing needed staffing for outpatient nutrition programs.

The second phase of our initiative is working outpatient RDs through the process of initiating programs or expanding their services. RDs in ARAMARK accounts will have a choice in their focus, either establishing a nutrition clinic where none has existed or developing a diabetes mellitus self-management training program (DMST) for their clients with diabetes mellitus. Some RDs may choose to work on both of these goals at the same time. RDs will be given templates for developing a business plan and a recognized DMST.

Benefits to participating ARAMARK client organizations will be increased revenues, including those from providing Medicare Part B MNT to patients with covered diagnoses, strengthened interdisciplinary collaboration, enhanced prominence of RDs in these facilities, and of course, positive patient outcomes.

Advanced-Level Practice: An Interview With Eve Callahan, RD, CNSD

Question: *Describe the work you do with patients.*

EVE CALLAHAN: My clinical practice is focused on providing the best nutrition care possible for the adult stem cell transplant

(SCT)/bone marrow transplant (BMT) patient population. Each patient is individually assessed for nutritional parameters prior to transplant. Patients and family are educated throughout the transplant process. Initially, education is provided on immunosuppression diet guidelines, food safety guidelines, individualized nutrient goals, and the use of diet records and calorie count forms.

As patients progress after transplant, they can have drug-induced renal insufficiency, steroid-induced diabetes mellitus, and graft-versus-host disease (GVHD). At this point, the education I provide is individualized to their needs and the progress they are making. Much time is spent in helping patients cope with the side effects of their chemotherapy and radiation therapy.

My day starts at 7:00 to 7:30 a.m. with preparation for BMT rounds: obtaining and assessing weights, vital signs, flow sheets, sliding-scale insulin requirements, labs, TPN [total parenteral nutrition] formulas, and the appropriateness of current diet orders. Calorie counts are reviewed with the dietetic technician, along with patients' food preferences for meals and snacks. Nutritional supplements are initiated, based on feedback provided by the dietetic technician.

From 8:00 to 9:30 a.m., I attend daily bedside rounds with the inpatient SCT/BMT team. Team rounds include the attending physician, the SCT/BMT pharmacist, two SCT/BMT nurse practitioners, the social worker, the SCT/BMT nurse case coordinator, and myself. I provide the team with patients' calorie count results, the contents of their current TPN regimens, and recommendations for changes in TPN that I feel are appropriate.

After rounds, I complete documentation in patients' medical records. This includes TPN notes and verbal orders for TPN. In addition, I revisit patients to provide education and discuss their nutrition concerns.

From 10:30 a.m. to 12:30 p.m., I see recently discharged SCT/BMT patients in the outpatient clinic and discuss their nutritional care with the outpatient SCT/BMT team. Most patients continue on calorie counts after discharge and need weekly follow-up on their home TPN and education on symptom management. Patients who are receiving outpatient SCT are also seen and educated. In addition to completing documentation, I contact patients' home care companies regarding updates on their TPN.

In the afternoons, I see patients on the SMT/BMT and hematology services, as needed. I also attend daily Nutrition Support Rounds and present to the team patients on my inpatient unit who are on TPN. In this capacity, I serve as the link between the SMT/BMT and Nutrition Support teams regarding patients' TPN.

Question: How does your work go beyond entry-level dietetic practice?

EC: I am a member of two multidisciplinary teams—the SCT/BMT and Nutrition Support teams. Many times on rounds, I get to educate other members of the teams on nutrition principals I have learned in my 12 years of experience working with these patients. I have been able to come into a newly created position at Vanderbilt University Medical Center and set up systems to help our program run better, in order to improve nutrition care for inpatients and outpatients.

Question: What advice would you give to other RDs who want to reach the level of advanced practice?
   EC:
   • Read everything you can on your area of practice. When I started in the area of SCT/BMT, I had been out of my internship for 2 months. I understood that I had to focus on learning everything about BMT/SCT and nutritional support.
   • Stay up-to-date on changes in nutrition care in areas that impact your practice or specialty by reading the professional literature. Every month, I read the *Journal of the American Dietetic Association, Nutrition in Clinical Practice, Journal of Parenteral and Enteral Nutrition,* and *Tufts Health and Nutrition Letter.* I read *Support Line,* the DNS newsletter quarterly. I also review evidence-based research on SCT/BMT using Ovid.
   • Be available and visible to your care team and, most importantly, to your patients. Communicate with your team about what you do for your patients. Be a patient advocate. Advocate to get issues addressed that you recognize as affecting your patients and their needs.
   • Talk and collaborate with peers in your specialty who work in other centers. Learn from their practices to make your systems better. Share your own best practices.
   • Obtain certification in your area of interest.

Advanced-Level Practice: An Interview With Ellen Ladage, RD, CNSD

Question: Describe the work you do with patients.
   ELLEN LADAGE: I work with patients on the general surgery unit and in the medical intensive care unit. In addition, I follow TPN patients and, until recently, was the liver transplant dietitian. I am currently working on setting up a care management program for our home tube feeding patients. The program will include patients who have been discharged on tube feedings, as well as those placed on tube feedings in the outpatient setting. Our goal with these patients is to ensure that nutrition goals are being met, needed resources are obtained, and complications are avoided. We will provide initial and follow-up consultation in our outpatient nutrition clinic, as well as telephonic monitoring and care.

Question: How does your work go beyond entry-level dietetic practice? (In other words, what about your work do you think makes it "advanced practice?")

EL: I work with complex patients—including critically ill medical patients, complex surgical patients, and those on complicated nutrition support regimens.

I try to work beyond minimum standards—to go the extra mile to provide the best possible nutrition care.

I strive to keep my knowledge up-to-date. I frequently read professional journals and literature, attend continuing education events, and maintain my certification as a nutrition support dietitian (CNSD). I wrote an article for a professional nursing journal this year. I serve as a resource person for others on the health care team and am a preceptor for dietetic interns.

I seek out ways to improve nutrition care provided at my hospital. Examples include writing and implementing the template for on-line documentation of medical nutrition therapy notes, revising and implementing the enteral formulary, and revising our evidence-based inpatient medical nutrition therapy protocols. I also evaluate and update patient education materials when needed.

Question: What would other RDs have to do to reach this level of advanced practice?

EL:
- Continue to learn . . . always.
- Be a resource person for others.
- Reach beyond the minimum standards to provide the best care possible.
- Seek out ways to improve the system.

REFERENCES

1. Nutrition Policy Task Force of the American Dietetic Association. *Discussion Paper on Food, Nutrition, and Health Policy.* March, 2002. Available at: http://www.eatright.com/images/leadership/nptf.pdf. Accessed May 13, 2003.
2. Fitzner K, Myers EF, Caputo N, Michael P. Are health plans changing their views on nutrition services coverage? *J Am Diet Assoc.* 2003;103:157–161.
3. Vinicor F. Population health and diabetes. *On the Cutting Edge.* 2003;24(1):4.
4. Wong F. RDs in population health. *On the Cutting Edge.* 2003;24(1):10–11.
5. Schiller MR, Arensberg MB, Kantor B. Administrator's perceptions of nutrition services in home health agencies. *J Am Diet Assoc.* 1998;98:55–61.
6. Sceery NL. Managing nutrition support in the home: integrating hospital and home care services. *Support Line* 2002;24:9–13,16.
7. Rosal MC, Ebberling CB, Lofgren I, Ockene JK, Hebert JR. Facilitating dietary change: the patient-centered counseling model. *J Am Diet Assoc.* 2001;101: 332–338, 341.
8. Barr JT, Schumacher GE. The need for a nutrition-related quality-of-life measure. *J Am Diet Assoc.* 2003;103:177–180.
9. The American Dietetic Association Foundation. Nutrition Quality of Life Tool. Available at: *http://www.bouve.neu.edu/nercoa.html.* Accessed October 12, 2003.
10. Institute of Medicine. *Dietary Reference Intakes for Calcium, Phosphorus, Magnesium, Vitamin D, and Fluoride.* Washington, DC: National Academy Press; 1997.

11. Institute of Medicine. *Dietary Reference Intakes for Thiamin, Riboflavin, Niacin, Vitamin B6, Folate, Vitamin B12, Pantothenic Acid, Biotin, and Choline*. Washington, DC: National Academy Press; 1998.

12. Institute of Medicine. *Dietary Reference Intakes for Vitamin C, Vitamin E, Selenium, and Carotenoids*. Washington, DC: National Academy Press; 2000.

13. Institute of Medicine. *Dietary Reference Intakes for Vitamin A, Vitamin K, Arsenic, Boron, Chromium, Copper, Iodine, Iron, Manganese, Molybdenum, Nickel, Silicon, Vanadium, and Zinc*. Washington, DC: National Academy Press; 2001.

14. Institute of Medicine. *Dietary Reference Intakes for Energy, Carbohydrate, Fiber, Fat, Fatty Acids, Cholesterol, Protein, and Amino Acids*. Washington, DC: National Academy Press; 2002.

15. Shattuck D. Nutritional genomics. *J Am Diet Assoc*. 2003;103:16–17.

16. Neighbors-Dembereckyj L, Painter JE. On-line diet analysis tools: a functional comparison. *J Am Diet Assoc*. 2002;102:1738–1742.

17. Key trends affecting the dietetics profession and the American Dietetic Association. *J Am Diet Assoc*. 2002;102(suppl):S1819-S1839.

18. Putnam RD. *Bowling Alone*. New York, NY: Simon and Schuster; 2000.

19. O'Sullivan Maillet J, Smith Edge M. Leading the future of dietetics. *J Am Diet Assoc*. 2003;103:420.

20. Parks SC. The fractured ant hill: a new architecture for sustaining the future. *J Am Diet Assoc*. 2002;102:33–38.

21. O'Sullivan Maillet J. Dietetics in 2017: what does the future hold? *J Am Diet Assoc*. 2002;102:1404–1406.

22. Franz MJ. The future of clinical dietetics: evidence, outcomes, and reimbursement. Lenna Frances Cooper Memorial Lecture, 2002 Food and Nutrition Exhibition and Conference, the American Dietetic Association; Philadelphia, Pa. October 23, 2002.

23. *2004 Hospital Accreditation Standards (HAS)*. Oakbrook Terrace, Ill: Joint Commission on Accreditation of Healthcare Organizations; 2004.

24. Myers EF, Barnhill G, Bryk J. Clinical privileges: missing piece of the puzzle for clinical standards that elevate responsibilities and salaries for registered dietitians? *J Am Diet Assoc*. 2002;102:123–132.

25. Moreland K, Gotfried M, Vaughn L. Development and implementation of the Clinical Privileges for Dietitian Nutrition Order Writing Program at a long-term acute-care hospital. *J Am Diet Assoc*. 2002;102:72–81.

CHAPTER 3

Developing a Staffing Plan

Differences in perceptions of clinical nutrition staffing needs may exist between administrators on the one hand and nutrition managers and clinical nutrition staff on the other. To maintain objectivity, administrators may rely on consultants to provide formulas or ratios of full-time equivalents (FTEs) per bed to use in calculating staffing needs. They also may rely on benchmarking data to ensure adherence to industry norms. Generally, administrators tend to focus on the financial impact of overstaffing rather than on the impact on the quality of nutrition care and patient outcomes resulting from understaffing, because relatively few data on the latter exist.

Nutrition managers and clinical nutrition staff are wise to view staffing from the perspective of their administrators, acknowledging the reality that these individuals want simple, consistent methods to predict staffing needs. Administrators trust the data in their financial reports to a greater extent than the data from patient care audits and internal nutrition department reports. They expect staffing plans that are within budget limitations and that meet patient needs, but do not exceed them. Administrators may define *best practice* differently than nutrition managers and clinical nutrition staff do.

The ability of a formula or ratio to predict staffing needs with accuracy depends on the quality of the process used to derive the model on which the calculations are based. The model should have a foundation in the professional literature. It should be validated through use in facilities similar to those of its intended use and should be current (ie, updated to reflect recent changes in health care).

Caution should accompany the use of staffing ratios from the literature that were not intended to be recommendations based on evidence, but rather were reports of existing staffing ratios. Examples are the ratios reported by Edelstein, Compher, and Colaizo for the Dietitians in Nutrition Support dietetic practice group (DPG), and by Scollard and Chima for the Clinical Nutrition Management DPG (1–3). These ratios are valuable in establishing norms at specific points in time, but they should not be used as the sole basis for predicting

STAFFING MODELS

staffing requirements. An example is the ratio of 1 registered dietitian (RD) to 100 beds reported by DNS in 1989 (2). Staffing models are described in the literature, and several models are outlined in the following sections.

Alford-Powers Model

The Alford-Powers model was developed by Margaret Alford-Powers, MPH, RD, a senior consultant with Dietary Management Advisory, Inc. A summary of the model was published in 1992 in *Future Dimensions,* the newsletter of the Clinical Nutrition Management DPG (4). Ranges of dietitian staffing were reported as FTEs per occupied bed by service (eg, 1/65 to 1/75 for a medical service and 1/30 to 1/60 for an intensive care unit). Staffing factors were derived from these ranges (eg, 0.013 to 0.017 dietitian FTE per occupied bed on a medical service and 0.017 to 0.033 dietitian FTE per occupied bed in an intensive care unit). The staffing factors were based on characteristics that affect expectations of care:

- Average length of stay
- Responsibility for completion of nutrition screening
- Patient acuity
- Type of medical service
- Availability of support staff
- Standards of care

The article reported the informal validation of this model at more than a dozen hospitals (4).

Department of Veterans Affairs Clinical Nutrition Staffing Model

The Department of Veterans Affairs (VA) Clinical Nutrition Staffing Model is based on the VA patient classification system that was described in Chapter 1. This model was reported in a 1998 issue of the *Journal of the American Dietetic Association* (5) and can be accessed online at http://*www.hsrd.ann-arbor.med.va.gov*/clinutstaf_jcl.htm (6).

Direct care time requirements have been established for total time per patient per category or group in the classification system and for types of nutrition activities within each category or group. The established time requirement is multiplied by the expected caseloads in each category or group to determine the direct care time requirement. This figure is added to the predicted indirect care and nonpatient time requirements to determine the total time requirement for dietitians.

Patient Acuity Staffing Study Model

The Patient Acuity Staffing Study (PAS) model began as a project of the Clinical Nutrition Management DPG that involved the collection of data at 92 acute care facilities during 1991 and 1992. Information on variables associated with medical nutrition therapy (MNT) time was collected, in addition to data on the time spent performing six common clinical tasks: nutrition screening, rescreening, intervention and documentation, intake analysis, counseling, and discharge planning.

The data were analyzed by Margaret Simmons, MS, RD, who used regression analysis to derive a formula for patient acuity time (PAT). MNT time for direct care can be calculated by sampling the facility's patient population, determining the nutritional acuity of the sampled population, calculating the PAT using the formula, and predicting MNT for the entire population. As with the VA Clinical Nutrition Staffing Model, with the PAS model total direct care time must be added to predicted indirect care time and nonpatient care time requirements to derive total requirements for dietitian time. The development of this model was reported in the September 1997 and Winter 1998 issues of *Future Dimensions in Clinical Nutrition Management*, although information on validation has not been reported (7,8).

Premier Clinical Benchmarking Tool

Approximately one in three hospitals belongs to the Premier purchasing group, an entity that promotes cost containment for its members through volume purchasing. The Premier Clinical Benchmarking Tool was developed by the group's Nutrition Task Force, a group composed of food service directors, clinical nutrition managers, and clinical dietitians selected from, and representative of, the member hospitals.

The Premier tool is used to determine the amount of time clinical dietitians spend in direct care and to make comparisons of time use—comparisons of individual facility performance over time and with performance of other facilities across the nation. This model assigns to direct care activities a specific number of allowed workload units (WLUs), or 15-minute increments of time. For example, a nutrition assessment in the inpatient setting is assigned 2 WLUs, or 30 minutes of time; a complex counseling session in the outpatient setting is assigned 4 WLUs, or 60 minutes of time (oral communication with Debra Kasper, RD, manager, clinical nutrition, Premier, Inc, May 2003).

WLU times calculated from this model can be compared with the activity time averages derived from facility audit data. Large deviations between measured activity times and activity times in the Premier tool may suggest errors in data collection.

Although the tool is not intended to be a model for predicting staffing needs, WLU assignments for direct care activities also can be used to determine the amount of dietitian time required for direct patient care, when used in conjunction with other audit data. For example, WLUs can be used with audit data on the number and type of activities required for nutrition care of patients at each level of nutritional risk to calculate an average direct care time requirement for patients at each nutritional risk level. Total direct care time requirements can be calculated by multiplying the calculated direct care time required at each nutritional risk level by the estimates of the projected numbers of patient admissions at each nutritional risk level, obtained from audit data.

The Premier tool does not assign WLUs to direct care activities based on patients' nutritional acuity. Therefore, if audit data reveal differences in time requirements to complete nutrition care activities at each nutritional risk level, the total time requirements calculated using only Premier WLUs may vary from calculations derived from more precise facility audit data. Still, they provide a valuable benchmark for comparison and a system to use until an audit can be completed.

DEPARTMENT-SPECIFIC STAFFING NEEDS

Nutrition Case Mix

To comply with the Joint Commission on Accreditation of Healthcare Organizations (JCAHO) human resources standards, nutrition departments are expected to define the case mix of the patients they serve, the types of nutrition care provided to patients with different levels of nutrition needs, and the staff needed to provide this care. The first step in this process is to determine the number of patients admitted to the facility who are at nutritional risk, by using the results of nutrition screening. In facilities that categorize patients into different levels of nutritional risk, numbers of patients at each level of nutritional risk need to be determined.

One way to obtain this information is to track the nutritional risk levels of all patients admitted to the facility over a specific interval of time (eg, a 1-month interval). Ideally, data are collected for more than one interval (eg, for a month during each quarter of the year). However, this system may not always be possible because of the time involved.

Another way to gather the needed information is to collect cross-sectional data or snapshots of the nutritional risk levels of hospitalized patients on several dates during the year, selecting a set of dates that provides a representative sampling of patients. Data are combined to give facility averages.

Both of these methods provide absolute numbers of patients at nutritional risk, as well as their relative proportions. The proportions can be applied to the total number of admissions for a 1-year interval to estimate numbers of patients admitted at each level of nutritional risk. Sample forms for both methods are in Appendixes C.1, C.2, and C.3. Completed examples of the first two forms are found in Appendixes D.1 and D.2.

Time Requirements for Nutrition Care Interventions

The next step in determining staffing needs is estimating or measuring the amount of clinical nutrition staff time required for general nutrition care activities (ie, the activities that are admission driven and/or

Factors That Affect Staffing Needs

- *Nutrition case mix:* the severity of nutritional risk of patients admitted to the facility
- *Patient volumes:* the numbers of admissions and average lengths of stay of patients at each level of nutritional risk
- *Time required for general patient care interventions:* nutrition screening, rescreening, determining nutritional risk level, and monitoring patients receiving nothing by mouth or clear liquids
- *Time required for direct nutrition care of patients at each nutritional risk level:* nutrition assessment, monitoring, reassessment, case management, and predischarge teaching
- *Average total direct care time for a patient at each level of nutritional risk*

result in the identification of patients needing individualized nutrition intervention). General nutrition care activities include nutrition screening, rescreening, evaluating nutritional risk status (ie, determining a patient's nutritional risk or priority level), and monitoring patients who are receiving nothing by mouth or only clear liquids. This step is followed by an estimation or measurement of the time requirements for direct nutrition care interventions (eg, nutrition assessment, monitoring, reassessment, case management activities, and predischarge teaching, for the average patient at each level of nutritional risk). The term used for the estimated or measured time to perform a nutrition care activity is its "activity factor."

The actual measurement of the use of time by staff during completion of their patient care activities over a defined time interval is generally more accurate than relying on estimates by staff, although the process takes considerable time and energy. One method is to have staff collect data while completing their own work. This method provides unit-specific data and time estimates, and it facilitates evaluation of workload distribution among staff. In addition, combined or aggregate data demonstrate staffing needs for the entire facility.

Accuracy and consistency of measurements are important. They are achieved by having written instructions, standard forms for use, and thorough training prior to data collection. It is also important to conduct a pilot study—either on one unit of the facility or, for a short time, on all units involved—prior to starting a full-scale time study, as well as to make revisions to the process and forms based on feedback received from the pilot study. Forms to use in a time study of general care, indirect and nonpatient care, and direct nutrition care activities are in Appendixes C.4 and C.5 (general care); Appendixes C.6 and C.7 (indirect and nonpatient care); and Appendixes C.8, C.9, and C.10 (direct nutrition care). See Appendixes D.3 through D.13 for completed examples of these forms.

Time Requirements for Patients at Different Levels of Nutritional Risk

To determine staffing needs, next measure the number and type of activities required for patients at each level of nutritional risk (ie, the typical care provided to patients at moderate and high nutritional risk). Although some facilities have this type of data in their computer databases, many do not. The time required to complete these activities can be determined by having staff use a separate set of "Direct Care Nutrition Audit" forms for patients at each level of nutritional risk to measure the types and amount of nutrition intervention required from admission to discharge. It may simplify the process to conduct audits for each nutritional risk level at different times (eg, for high-risk patients one month and for moderate-risk patients the next month).

If staff time is limited, an alternate option is to ask staff to estimate these care requirements based on the average length of stay for each nutritional risk level. For example, staff might estimate that a typical patient at high nutritional risk receives an initial nutrition assessment and two reassessments during hospitalization. The total time for direct nutrition care can be estimated by using the average activity times (ie, the activity factors) from the measurement of direct care activity requirements or by using WLUs (eg, WLUs from the Premier model). (Example: Initial assessment = 30 minutes + 2 reassessments, each 15 minutes = 60 minutes average total nutrition care time for a patient admitted at high nutritional risk.)

Impact. It is important to collect data, even if a decision has been made to use an existing staffing model, in order to establish a baseline for future comparisons. The availability of data also facilitates determination of areas where changes are needed.

However, time studies have their limitations. They carry the assumption that staff members are performing work in the same manner during data collection as they would under normal circumstances. This assumption may or may not be true and should be taken into consideration. The amount of time spent on nutrition care activities will vary among individual staff members. And actual time spent on nutrition care may not be the same as desired time; staff may spend either too much or too little time on specific activities. Although these factors cannot be eliminated, they can be minimized by averaging the data collected from all staff members and by evaluating patient outcomes and other performance data, not just volumes of activities completed.

As an example of how to use both activity and outcome data, say recent aggregate outcome data indicate that patients are not achieving the goals defined in their nutrition care plans. One factor to consider would be the adequacy of the time the staff members have for nutrition assessment and monitoring. If patients are not achieving their goals, it may be because staff members are unable to thoroughly assess the causes of identified nutrition problems because of the time required to interview patients and investigate in the depth needed. If this is the case, the nutrition interventions they implement may not target the correct sources of nutrition problems, leading to problem continuation rather than resolution. Or staff members may lack time for frequent patient monitoring, resulting in a lack of timely adjustments in nutrition care plans. With sufficient time for reviewing patient data, the staff members would have noted that their interventions were not producing the intended results, and they would have made the required adjustments.

Determining Total Patient Nutrition Care Time Requirements

Overall projections of total hours of staff time needed for patient care are determined by adding the total time required for general nutrition care for all patients and the time required for direct nutrition care for patients at each level of nutritional risk (total direct patient nutrition care time). Determinations of total direct patient nutrition care time are made by multiplying the estimated numbers of patients admitted to the facility each year at each level of nutritional risk by the measurements or estimates of time required for direct care at each risk level (see Appendix C.11, "Patient Care Staffing Estimates" and Appendix D.14 for a completed example of that form). For example, if the average patient at high nutritional risk at a facility requires 60 minutes of direct care time, and 1,000 high-risk patients are admitted to the facility each year (assuming 25% of admissions are high risk and 4,000 total admissions per year), 1,000 hours of RD time is needed to provide direct care for these patients.

> **Total Patient Nutrition Care Time**
>
> Total patient nutrition care time is the *sum* of the following:
>
> - Time required for general patient nutrition care
> - Average total direct care time for each nutritional risk level × the number of patients admitted per year at each nutritional risk level (= total direct patient nutrition care time)

Determining Total Staffing Needs

The next step is to measure or estimate indirect nutrition care activities (eg, team rounds and care conferences) and nonpatient care and other activities (eg, student training, community presentations, staff monitoring, performance improvement activities, and evaluations). Total patient care time is added to estimates of the time required for indirect patient care activities, nonpatient care activity time, and nonproductive time (eg, vacations, holidays, and educational leave) to obtain the requirement for total staff hours. The total number of hours from this calculation is converted to FTEs by dividing by 2,080 (1 FTE = 2,080 hours). The process of converting FTEs to a staffing plan and work schedules is described later in the chapter.

> **Total Clinical Staff Hours Required**
>
> Total clinical staff hours needed is the *sum* of the following:
>
> - Total patient care time
> - Indirect care time
> - Nonpatient care time
> - Nonproductive time (eg, vacations, holidays, and education leave)

Estimating Outpatient Staffing Needs

Estimation of staffing needs in the outpatient setting can be challenging, in part because in many clinics, the no-show rate is high. In other words, a substantial number of patients make appointments but do not keep them or notify the office of a need to reschedule their appointments. Some clinic managers prefer to compensate for these patients by limiting or omitting the amount of indirect time included in their outpatient staffing estimates. They ask staff to complete indirect activities, such as documentation, dietary analyses, and program planning, during the times of the no-show appointments.

Appendix C.12 contains a form for estimating outpatient staffing needs. In using this form, managers should estimate the volume of expected outpatients by diagnosis and multiply these numbers by the time requirements for individual counseling for each diagnosis that were derived from the MNT Protocols and MNT Guides of the ADA (9–11). Managers also need to measure or estimate time requirements for other types of patients and any group sessions. Total time requirements are derived by combining estimates of total patient care time with calculated needs for vacation and relief coverage and indirect time, if included. Appendix D.15 shows a completed example of this form.

The forms for completing a thorough time study to measure staffing needs are found in Appendixes C.4 through C.11. Although the forms may need some modifications to individualize them according to facility needs, they provide the tools that managers and staff can use to determine their staffing needs. Facilities probably will need to use estimates to determine a portion of their staffing needs because of lack of needed data and the amount of time that actual measurements entail. Benchmarking with other facilities provides valuable feedback on whether or not estimates are realistic.

STAFFING PLAN The rest of this chapter describes how to aggregate the facility-specific information discussed in Chapter 1 and the data collected using the methods just described into a staffing plan that meets existing needs for clinical nutrition services.

The data that have been collected through time studies or careful estimations of time requirements can be used to calculate the number of FTEs needed by a nutrition department. These FTEs must be converted into actual positions and a staffing plan.

When developing a staffing plan, one of the first issues to explore is distribution of the clinical FTEs (ie, whether to have an all-dietitian staff or to include a combination of dietitians and dietetic technicians). This decision depends on several factors and will require the use of facility-specific data on volume of nutrition interventions for patients at low and moderate nutritional risk and the amount of time required for these interventions. The calculated FTEs for this work can be allocated to dietetic technicians, assuming that no state regulations limit the scope of practice to RDs. In addition, some indirect and nonpatient care activities can be assigned to dietetic technicians.

A small facility may not have sufficient volume to support both a full-time dietitian and a full-time dietetic technician. Facilities in this situation have several options, including having only a full-time dietitian or having a combination of full- and part-time staff. In small facilities, it is often possible for clinical staff to assume food service management duties so that full-time hours can be justified.

Another consideration in distributing FTEs, and often a major one, is the availability of dietetic technicians, especially dietetic technicians, registered (DTRs). Information included in the report of the 1999 ADA Member Database, which had a 77.3% response rate, indicated that hospitals and acute care facilities are the largest employment setting for DTRs (41.3%). However, the absolute number of DTRs employed is small (612 DTRs) when compared with the large number of health care facilities in this country. (12) In other words, DTRs may not be available, even though a need for their services can be supported with data.

This situation has led many facilities to use non-DTR dietetic technicians who work under the oversight or supervision of RDs ultimately responsible for patient care. Qualifications required for non-DTR dietetic technicians are facility specific, although it is not uncommon for facilities to require a college degree with nutrition course work. Some facilities have hired individuals who completed the course requirements for dietetic registration but did not obtain placement in dietetic internships.

Once the decision about distribution of clinical FTEs has been made, this information can be summarized in written form and used for comparisons with actual and budgeted staffing levels. Appendix C.13 contains a sample summary form.

Compare Calculations With Budget

Before proceeding further, it is wise to compare the calculated FTEs with budgeted FTEs (see Table 3.1). If the calculations and budgeted numbers are similar, from an organizational perspective, the plan is in alignment. If the numbers are different, the reason for variation needs to be identified. Variation may be due to having accurate calculations, but ones that are in excess of realistic expectations for numbers of staff. A way to determine if this is the case is to benchmark calculations with an existing staffing model. Benchmarking allows comparisons of calculated FTE needs with the needs derived from the model or models selected. Some benchmarking programs also allow comparison with staffing levels in other, similar facilities.

If FTE calculations and benchmark data agree, it is possible that the budgeted numbers are too low to meet patients' needs for nutrition care. When this is the case, the facility can take steps to obtain a change in budgeted numbers—that is, add staff.

However, if budgeted numbers and benchmark data agree, but are different from calculated FTEs, needs for optimal nutrition care would appear to be higher than the budget will allow and higher than the staffing norms reported via benchmarking. This discrepancy is possible because few data are available on either the outcomes of nutrition

Table 3.1   Evaluating the Numbers

Calculated staffing needs can be evaluated by comparisons with budgeted staffing and benchmark levels.

Calculations	Budgeted Numbers	Benchmark Numbers	Possible Explanations
Agree	Agree	Agree	There is alignment of numbers.
Agree	Disagree	Agree	Budgeted numbers may be too low to meet needs. Consider increasing the staffing budget.
Disagree	Agree	Agree	This finding may indicate a need for more staff because of facility-specific factors. Justification is required.

intervention in the acute care setting or the impact of different levels of staffing on the quality of nutrition intervention. Justification for additional staffing would need to be supported by strong facility-specific data collected during monitoring of nutrition intervention and staffing effectiveness to convince administrators of the necessity of adding staff. See Chapter 5 for an in-depth discussion of this topic.

Finalize Staffing Needs

By now, the manager should have a good understanding of FTE needs for dietitians and dietetic technicians. Before proceeding, it's wise to recheck calculations, especially calculations for nonproductive time (ie, vacation and relief coverage). Once calculations have been rechecked and the numbers of staff needed verified, the next step is creation of a schedule template. Making a template takes the entire process to the practical level and allows managers to evaluate whether the calculations derived actually provide the coverage that is needed.

If an existing schedule template is available, it can be used. If a template is not available, one should be created. (Refer to the sample schedule template in Appendix C.14.) The template should cover a relatively short period (eg, a 1-week or 2-week period). It should list all units or areas to be covered, as well as positions listed by number rather than by the name of the staff member. Creating a template requires careful thought and consideration about the appropriate unit assignments for each position listed. Input from current staff can be helpful in ensuring that coverage is adequate and realistic.

Once the schedule template is made, a rotation for weekend coverage is needed. Like the template, the weekend rotation should include areas of coverage and position numbers. Staffing should be adequate to meet the time standards established for completing nutrition care activities, as defined in JCAHO standards and department policies and procedures.

A separate template schedule and weekend rotation is needed for each group of dietitians in a rotation cluster. For example, at a facility with separate dietitians for adult and pediatric patients, templates and weekend schedules are needed for both the dietitians assigned to adult units and the dietitians assigned to pediatric units. In this example, it may be possible to link the weekend rotations of the dietitians by having cross-coverage. However, this option should be available only when both groups of dietitians have demonstrated competencies in all areas of coverage.

Once the template and the weekend rotation have been created, sample schedules can be developed. The number of sample schedules should cover an interval that allows the entire weekend rotation to elapse. This method ensures weekday coverage for days off for working weekends. For example, if the schedule template includes six dietitians, and one dietitian works each weekend, 6 weeks of sample schedules will be needed for a cycle of the entire weekend rotation.

Sometimes calculations that seem right do not appear to meet needs. When this happens, adjustments may be needed. If identified staffing needs have been well thought out, any needed adjustments should be minor.

Templates can be more difficult to plan when dietitians have cross-coverage in both inpatient and outpatient areas. In these circumstances, clinic coverage will need to be incorporated into the template. Backup coverage of inpatient areas may be needed while staff members are working in outpatient clinics, and days off for weekend coverage will need to be assigned with clinic coverage in mind.

Adherence to the Staffing Plan

The final component of assessing staff adequacy is an evaluation of how close actual FTEs and work schedules are to projections of needs. This evaluation involves a comparison of data on worked and paid time for staff, obtained from budget reports, with calculated staffing needs (Appendix C.13). This comparison can be made by month, quarter, and year. Another way to evaluate staffing adequacy is to calculate the number and percentage of days with full staffing according to the staffing plan. Chapter 5 describes the assessment of staffing effectiveness in detail.

REFERENCES

1. Edelstein SF. Staffing and fee levels for clinical nutrition services in pediatric hospitals in the United States and Canada. *J Am Diet Assoc.* 1991;91:1991.
2. Compher C, Colaizo T. Staffing patterns in hospital clinical dietetics and nutrition support: a survey conducted by the Dietitians in Nutrition Support Dietetic Practice Group of the American Dietetic Association. *J Am Diet Assoc.* 1992;92:807–812.
3. Scollard TM, Chima C. 1999 CNM staffing survey: summary of results. *Future Dimensions in Clinical Nutrition Management.* 2002;21(4):1–5.
4. Alford-Powers M. Clinical nutrition services staffing. *Future Dimensions in Clinical Nutrition Management.* 1992;11(1):5–8.
5. Shavink-Dillerud M, Lowery J, Striplin D. Development of clinical nutrition staffing model. *J Am Diet Assoc.* 1998;98(suppl):A23.
6. Department of Veterans Affairs. VA Clinical Nutrition Staffing Model. Available at: http://*www.hsrd.ann-arbor.med.va.gov*/clinutstaf_jcl.htm. Accessed October 12, 2003.
7. Simmons ML. Patient acuity staffing study, I. *Future Dimensions in Clinical Nutrition Management.* 1997;16(4):1–4, 6.
8. Simmons ML. Patient acuity staffing study, II: the medical nutrition therapy model and applications. *Future Dimensions in Clinical Nutrition Management.* 1998;17(1):12–17, 20.
9. *American Dietetic Association Medical Nutrition Therapy Evidence-Based Guides for Practice* [CD-ROMs]. Chicago, Ill: American Dietetic Association; 2002.
10. American Dietetic Association and Morrison Health Care. *Medical Nutrition Therapy Across the Continuum of Care: Supplement 1.* Chicago, Ill: American Dietetic Association; 1997.

11. American Dietetic Association and Morrison Health Care. *Medical Nutrition Therapy Across the Continuum of Care.* 2nd ed. Chicago, Ill: American Dietetic Association; 1998.
12. Dietetic Practice Audit Panels of 1997–98, 1998–99, and 1999–2000 of the Commission on Dietetic Registration. 2000 Commission on Dietetic Registration dietetics practice audit. *J Am Diet Assoc.* 2002;102:270–292.

CHAPTER 4

Implementing a Staffing Plan and New Clinical Programs

O nce a staffing plan has been developed, it has to be implemented. Implementation may involve adjustments in staffing—either additions when new programs are initiated and services are expanded, or reductions when programs are eliminated or streamlined. On a smaller scale, implementation may involve the transition of staff from one program or care setting to another. It also may involve refining daily workflow and care processes or initiating the collection of data needed for monitoring outcomes and staffing effectiveness. Implementation is the "do" of the plan-do-check-act performance improvement cycle, and it is a critical stage linking careful planning with desired results.

This chapter discusses key factors to address in the implementation process. It also discusses issues specific to staffing that may arise during the transitions that occur with implementation.

Change involves people. And whereas there are always those people who jump at the chance for change, many are slower in accepting the need for change and taking the steps to accomplish it. This reality of the work world reflects the fact that change in one area affects many other areas of work life because of the complex interactions among staff and patient care processes.

Involve Staff Affected by the Change

Involving staff in the change process is useful for many reasons. First, staff members bring insight and information from different perspectives, and this insight can be incorporated into the design of the new processes and programs. In other words, the final processes and programs will be of higher quality because of the involvement of staff members. Second, it is essential to build the trust of staff in new programs and processes, and this trust is born, in part, from their involvement in the changes that affect their jobs and daily routines. Staff

IMPLEMENTATION OVERVIEW

CHALLENGE OF CHANGE

Resources for Managing Change

Biesemeier C, Schofield M, Marino L. *Connective Leadership: Linking Vision with Action.* Chicago, Ill: American Dietetic Association; 2001.

Bridges W. *Managing Transitions: Making the Most of Changes.* Reading, Mass: Addison-Wesley; 1991.

Collins J. *Good to Great: Why Some Companies Make the Leap—and Others Don't.* New York, NY: HarperCollins; 2001.

Katzenbach J, Smith D. *The Wisdom of Teams.* Boston, Mass: McKinsey; 1994.

Winer M, Ray K. *Collaboration Handbook: Creating, Sustaining, and Enjoying the Journey.* St Paul, Minn: Amherst H. Wilder Foundation; 1994.

members already have been involved in the planning process, if the time studies described in Chapter 3 were completed. Now it is time to expand their involvement.

In small departments, it may be possible to include all affected staff on what could be called the change team. However, most of the time it is necessary to build a team that includes representatives from the different levels of staff. Depending on the nature of the change, teams also may include representatives from different departments. In any case, team members are responsible for ongoing and two-way communication with the groups they represent.

Teams start out as groups of individuals brought together for a common task. To be effective, the individuals on teams must unite in their efforts. Effective teamwork takes time and energy to achieve.

Build Acceptance of the Change

Even when staff members have been involved in identifying the need for change and in defining the direction of the changes that are occurring, the reality of change at its actual implementation can be much different from the energized discussions of the planning process. Once a change team is formed, team leaders need to ensure that team members understand the work they are undertaking.

As William Bridges says in his book *Managing Transitions,* one way to build acceptance is to sell the problem, not the solution (1). In other words, staff members need to review and completely understand the data that were collected and analyzed in the initial planning stages. They need to explore the issues created by staffing imbalances and the impact these imbalances have on department operation. They also need to define the impact on themselves individually, as well as on the groups they represent; they need to ask, What's in it for me? Only when staff members perceive that there is a problem and a need to change will they be willing to offer their full support. Appendix E.1 contains an activity that teams can use to define existing problems and the benefits of proposed changes. Box 4.1 is an example of how this form can be used by a team.

Develop Implementation Plans

Implementation plans are the detailed listings of steps, accountabilities, and time lines for the projects that are included in the strategic plan. Implementation plans are also developed for projects and activities outside the strategic plan that must be completed. Unlike the strategic plan, an implementation plan very clearly defines who does what, and when. Both types of plans are important to department operation, just as on a trip, both an itinerary and a road map are needed for travel from one point to the next.

Box 4.1 Team Activity: Evaluating the Impact of Changes

Proposed Change: *Expansion in DTR hours in a pediatric hospital.*

List problems or unmet needs that exist as a result of the current situation:

1. *RDs spend large amounts of time on activities that a DTR could do (eg, determining food preferences and menu selection with oncology patients).*

2. *Calorie counts for pediatric oncology and BMT patients are not completed until late morning.*

What problems does the current situation create for the work group I represent?

1. *RDs don't have enough time to see pediatric oncology outpatients.*

2. *Calorie count data are not available in time for morning pediatric oncology rounds. This creates a delay in making decisions about nutrition support.*

List three benefits or positive aspects of implementing the proposed program or staffing plan for the unit as a whole:

1. *Expansion of RD role with pediatric oncology outpatients.*

2. *Improved patient care.*

3. *Potential for increased revenue from billable RD services.*

How will these changes benefit the work group that I represent?

1. *Enhanced role of RD on the pediatric oncology team.*

2. *Increased RD job satisfaction.*

One method that change teams can use to develop an implementation plan is gap analysis. This method involves developing specific answers to three questions:

1. *Desired status:* Where do we want to be when we have met the objective and completed the project?

2. *Current status:* Where are we now?
3. *Action steps:* What will it take to get us from where we are now to where we want to be?

Gap Analysis

Gap analysis focuses on three key questions:

1. Where do we want to be?
2. Where are we now?
3. What do we have to do to get from where we are now to where we want to be?

The action steps that are developed in answer to the third question should include deadlines for completion of each step and specific accountabilities—that is, the names of the individuals responsible for each action step. Structural or process changes, resource needs, and methods of communication should be identified. As with any project, it is important to allow enough time for completion of the action steps, without extending the project over such a long period that momentum is lost. Appendix E.2 is a form that can be used for completing a gap analysis and developing an implementation plan for a project. Figure 4.1 demonstrates how an implementation form can be used.

Problem-Solving Approach to Barriers

Barriers are the factors that stand in the way of success—in this case, in the way of implementing plans for staffing, developing and initiating new nutrition programs and services, and refining existing programs and services. Some barriers can be anticipated; others arise unexpectedly.

Part of the process of developing an implementation plan is identifying actual and potential barriers to carrying out the steps in the plan and determining the best approach to their resolution. The evaluation process that occurs as a result may lead to refinements in the original implementation plan. The best solutions often arise after the team has brainstormed to identify several possible resolution strategies and has considered the merits of each strategy. Regular team meetings offer a good opportunity to assess progress in implementing the plans that have been made. These gatherings are also a good time to identify new barriers to meeting project deadlines that have arisen and to develop strategies to overcome them. See Box 4.1 for an example of how a team evaluates the impact of changes. Appendix E.3 contains a tool that teams can use to overcome barriers in this problem-solving process, and Box 4.2 and Box 4.3 show examples of this form as it could be completed.

COMMON ISSUES   Decisions about how to make staffing changes are reflected in the strategies defined in the implementation plan. Staffing changes can be made relatively rapidly, by moving staff in existing positions to needed positions. In contrast, the changes can be made more slowly, through attrition and hiring replacements into the new positions. Attrition may be a reasonable option when it is anticipated at the time the implementation plan is developed. However, if attrition is not expected to

Performance Area	Strategies	Due Date	Responsibility	Progress
Internal Processes				
RD duties	1. Meet with RD to discuss changes in daily routines and feasibility of changing normal work hours.	2/05	CNM	
DTR duties	1. Outline daily duties and work flow.	2/05	CNM & RD	
	2. Develop job description.	2/05	CNM	
	3. Write policies and procedures related to calorie counts as needed.	5/05	RD	
	4. Hire DTR.	6/05	CNM w/RD input	
	Completion Date			
Finances				
Budget	1. Prepare proposal with justification for adding a 0.5 FTE DTR.	3/05	CNM	
	2. Meet with department director to review proposal, identify additional information/data needed for approval, and select implementation date.	4/05	CNM	
	3. Contact benefits coordinators to discuss MNT coverage for outpatient pediatric oncology patients.	5/05	CNM & RD	
	Completion Date			
Customers				
Needs of pediatric oncology outpatient staff—define RD role	1. Meet with outpatient clinic manager and MD director to determine needs, explore potential RD roles, and develop time frame for implementation.	1/05	CNM	
	2. Meet with clinic staff to identify types of patients needing RD intervention and specific nutrition needs of patients.	1/05	CNM & RD	
	Completion Date			

Figure 4.1 Implementation plan. See Appendix E.2 for template.

Figure 4.1 (*continued*)

Performance Area	Strategies	Due Date	Responsibility	Progress
Innovation and Learning				
RD duties	*1. Communicate with other RDs with similar roles via contacts within Pediatric Nutrition Practice Group.*	*2/05*	*RD*	
	2. Obtain and review reference materials.	*2/05–4/05*	*RD*	
	3. Schedule training with outpatient pediatric oncology staff.	*6/05*	*RD*	
DTR duties	*1. Perform department and job-specific training subsequent to hiring.*	*7/05*	*RD*	
	2. Have pediatric oncology RD explain policies and pro-cedures and other unit-specific information.	*7/05*	*RD*	
	Completion Date			

occur in a reasonably short time, it is better to actively make the changes.

Some changes in staffing can be implemented without the involvement of the human resources department—for example, when no changes in the number and grade of positions will occur. Other changes will require the involvement of the human resources department; an example is adding or eliminating positions, particularly when an occupied position will be eliminated. Human resources departments usually have specific procedures that must be followed to ensure equity and fairness from a legal perspective.

The implementation of changes in staffing plans and staff assignments is not the time for taking actions needed because of poor performance. Any performance issues should be handled separately, and managers should follow the procedures for progressive discipline established by the human resources department. Combining performance management actions with the implementation of staffing-related changes will be apparent to staff and will contribute to feelings of distrust.

Staff members who are making changes in positions and job duties may not have the competencies needed for their new roles. Training should be provided when needed to ensure that staff members have the required knowledge and skills. For staff members in transition from the inpatient to the outpatient setting, the *American Dietetic Association Medical Nutrition Therapy Evidence-Based Guides for Practice*

Box 4.2   Overcoming Barriers: Example of a Large-Group Activity

Large-Group Activity: List the barriers that will need to be addressed when implementing the proposed changes.

Actual Barriers

1. *The current DTR daily routine is full—has no time for additional duties.*

2. *Changes are needed in the FTE budget and the salary and benefits budget to add a part-time DTR.*

3. *Need to determine the willingness of the outpatient pediatric oncology clinic to have an RD work with patients.*

4. *The RD needs training on outpatient clinic procedures.*

5. *The RD's work schedule needs to change to an earlier time frame to allow prep time for daily inpatient team rounds.*

6. *A space is needed where the outpatient RD will see patients.*

Potential Barriers

1. *Potential lack of reimbursement for MNT for pediatric oncology patients.*

Box 4.3   Overcoming Barriers: Example of a Small-Group Activity

Small-Group Activity: Divide into groups of two or three people. Assign one actual barrier to each small group.

Barrier: *Reluctance of outpatient pediatric oncology clinic staff to have an RD work with patients.*

List ways to resolve the barrier. Specify actions to be taken and persons responsible for taking actions.

1. *Meet with the outpatient clinic manager and the MD director to determine needs, explore the potential RD role, and develop a time frame for implementation.*

2. *Meet with clinic staff to identify the types of patients needing RD intervention and specific nutrition needs of patients.*

3. *Have the RD shadow two or three nurses, observe clinic operation, identify appropriate times and location for meeting with patients, build relationships with staff, and obtain training on procedures.*

4. *Develop a schedule template for patient appointments with the RD.*

are a good resource (2). A review of their content provides an update on disease-specific MNT for the outpatient setting. Continuing professional education credits are available for individuals who review each guide.

Change involves people, and people respond better to a systematic process than to a random or haphazard one. Thus, managers need to promote orderliness in the change process. Staff members are usually expected to complete their daily nutrition care activities while changes are being implemented. Therefore, managers must consider the staff members' time limits. Managers also need to plan stress relievers—events that are fun and allow staff members time to unwind together. Finally, there should be an end to the cycle of change. Achieving an ending can be difficult, because new cycles of change may overlap the current one. However, staff members will appreciate knowing that a particular phase or project has ended.

REFERENCES   1. Bridges W. *Managing Transitions: Making the Most of Changes*. Reading, Mass: Addison-Wesley; 1991.
2. *American Dietetic Association Medical Nutrition Therapy Evidence-Based Guides for Practice* [CD-ROMs]. Chicago, Ill: American Dietetic Association; 2002.

CHAPTER 5

Measuring and Evaluating Staffing Effectiveness

By now, a well-designed staffing plan has been formulated, using the information in Chapter 1 to assess staffing needs and the material in Chapter 3 to develop the plan. The plan has been refined to meet staffing needs for new and expanded programs, as discussed in Chapter 2. And it has been implemented, using strategies outlined in Chapter 4. The next phase of the performance improvement cycle for staffing is checking or studying the impact of implementation of the staffing plan to determine how well needs for patient care are being met.

At times, the evaluation or assessment processes can seem overwhelming to managers and staff. With the many demands on time that exist, it can be tempting to implement a plan and make changes to it on an as-needed basis, in response to emerging needs. However, as noted in Chapter 1, the Joint Commission on Accreditation of Healthcare Organizations (JCAHO) standards require that facilities provide an adequate number of staff members who have qualifications that are matched to their job responsibilities. To know whether this requirement has been met, projections for staffing needs must be compared with actual staffing levels, and variances must be identified and used to refine the staffing plan.

It is important to distinguish this type of evaluation—the evaluation of staffing needs and the use of the staffing plan—from other types of evaluations that managers perform to evaluate department performance, such as analysis of productivity and revenues and evaluation of staffing effectiveness. All three types of evaluations are important and are discussed in this chapter. Forms for collecting and summarizing performance data are included in Appendix F, including the "Annual Performance Tracking" form (Appendix F.1) and the "Summary Performance Report" (Appendix F.2).

EVALUATION OF ACTUAL STAFFING COMPARED WITH PLAN

The first type of evaluation involves determining whether the staffing plan is being used as it was intended. This evaluation involves a comparison of actual schedules with the staffing plan and a determination of variances. Comparisons can be made for a set of schedules both as they were planned (ie, before they were actually worked) and after they were actually worked. The number of schedules selected for comparison should be representative of overall staffing, for example, a month each year or 2 weeks each quarter. Comparisons can be made manually, in which case a smaller number of schedules may be evaluated. Or managers can create automated schedule spreadsheets that allow all schedules to be compared with the staffing plan. Forms for use in evaluating staffing plan compliance are included in Appendixes F.3 and F.4.

Initially, this type of comparison may seem unnecessary. However, unlike the ideal situations that are envisioned when plans are developed, real-life staffing issues arise frequently and make adherence to plans challenging. In addition, the timing of variance provides useful information. For example, variance between planned schedules and the staffing plan may indicate one of several things: a difference between the desired staffing plan and the number of approved positions on the schedule; vacancies in approved positions due to turnover or extended leaves; or an excess number of staff members taking paid vacation leave at the same time, pointing to a potential need for tighter policies on requests for, and approval of, vacations. Although sometimes unavoidable, shortages in planned schedules do not allow flexibility for unexpected events. Variances in worked schedules, but not planned schedules, indicate a tendency for staff members to take unplanned leave, such as sick time.

The data by themselves do not indicate causes of problems, although data on the amount and frequency of unplanned leave help indicate the extent of a problem, if one exists. Managers and staff can work together, using the data collected, to identify problems, their root causes, and solutions to implement.

EVALUATING DEPARTMENT PERFORMANCE

The second type of evaluation involves assessment of the results of department work (ie, the type and amount of work performed, or productivity); factors that affect productivity (eg, absenteeism and turnover); and the impact of the work (eg, customer satisfaction and staff satisfaction). This section describes methods for evaluating department performance. As will be explained later, the selection and evaluation of a set of these performance indicators is the basis for a staffing effectiveness evaluation program and for participation in facility-wide staffing effectiveness initiatives.

Productivity

Productivity is defined as the "ratio of the quantity and quality of units produced to the labor per unit of time" (1). Practically speaking, *productivity* is a term used to indicate how well staff members use their time to accomplish the work that needs to be done. It can be measured in several ways.

Activity Volumes and Revenues

One way to measure productivity is to compare actual volumes of activities performed with projected numbers obtained from the annual budget. Generally, monthly volume totals are used for comparison, as are year-to-date totals. In addition, current-year volumes and volumes of prior years can be compared.

To do this type of monitoring, a tracking system is needed. The system can be either manual or automated. Data from both manual and automated systems are usually self-reported. However, sophisticated automated systems can capture and aggregate data from on-line documentation programs. (Refer to Appendixes F.5, F.6, and F.7 for forms that staff can use to track and summarize the volume of activities completed.)

Data accuracy depends on clear delineation of activities being tracked, in order to avoid reporting the same activities in more than one category or omitting some activities altogether. The accuracy of data also depends on the appropriate and sensitive use of the data gathered by managers, in order to encourage accurate reporting by staff.

For legitimate reasons, variation in activity volumes from one unit to another may lead to variation in individual performance. For example, a dietitian on a general medicine—surgery unit might well report higher volumes of nutrition assessments than a dietitian working in an intensive care unit because of the need for more in-depth nutrition assessment in the intensive care unit. However, if staff members believe they will be held accountable for completing the same amount of work as their peers, regardless of the existence of legitimate factors that result in lower numbers, they will have the incentive to exaggerate their volumes and overestimate work performed.

For this reason, it is often preferable to emphasize aggregate numbers when sharing data with staff, upper-level managers, and administrators. Sharing individual data can be reserved for performance evaluations (eg, comparing total volumes of work accomplished from one year to the next).

Another type of productivity evaluation is the comparison of actual revenues with budgeted revenues. As with activity volumes, several comparisons usually are made (ie, comparisons by month, as year to date, and with prior years). Revenue volumes are derived from administrative reports that capture revenues from manual or automated billing systems. Forms to use in tracking activity and revenue volumes are located in Appendix F. See Figure 5.1 through 5.5 for examples of completed forms from Appendixes F.6 through F.10.

Impact. Evaluation of activity volumes and revenues provides an assessment of compliance with the annual budget—that is, whether or not the actual volumes of activities and revenues are at, above, or below budgeted levels. Any variance must be explained by exploring

RD ___ CD ___

Dates	Nutrition Screening	Nutrition Assessment: MR	Nutrition Assessment: HR	Nutrition Diagnosis: Weight Loss*	Nutrition Diagnosis: Inadequate Intake*	Reassessment MR	Reassessment: HR	Calorie Counts HR	Calorie Counts MR	Basic Education HR	Basic Education MR	Complex Education HR	Complex Education MR
Monday 10-6	0	2	10	8	8	1	2	1	0	2	1	2	0
Tuesday 10-7	0	1	8	8	8	2	4	1	0	1	0	0	0
Wednesday 10-8	0	1	8	6	6	0	4	2	0	0	1	1	0
Thursday 10-9	0	2	10	8	7	0	3	1	0	2	2	2	1
Friday 10-10	0	1	7	5	7	1	5	1	0	3	1	1	0
Saturday 10-11	—	—	—	—	—	—	—	—	—	—	—	—	—
Sunday 10-12	—	—	—	—	—	—	—	—	—	—	—	—	—
Totals	0	7	43	35	36	4	18	6	0	8	2	6	1

Figure 5.1 Completed Direct Care Activity Tracking Form (with nutrition diagnoses)

Abbreviations: HR, high risk; MR, moderate risk. — indicates no data collected.

*List the number of patients who received high-risk nutrition assessment and who had a nutrition diagnosis of weight loss and/or inadequate intake. List patients with both nutrition diagnoses in both columns. These numbers will provide an overall estimate of the relative proportions of high-risk patients with these two nutrition diagnoses.

Instructions:

1. List the number of each activity performed by date. List the total number of each activity completed for the week in the last row.
2. Transfer the totals to the "Direct Care Activity Individual Summary" form (Appendix F.7).

Name   _CD_

Month   _October_

Dates	Nutrition Screening	Nutrition Assessment: MR	Nutrition Assessment: High Risk (HRA)	Reassessment MR	Reassessment HR	Calorie Counts HR	Calorie Counts MR	Basic Education HR	Basic Education MR	Complex Education HR	Complex Education MR
10-1 to 10-3	0	2	27	3	2	1	0	2	2	2	1
10-6 to 10-10	0	7	43	4	18	6	0	8	2	6	1
10-13 to 10-17	5	10	38	8	12	8	2	7	6	5	2
10-20 to 10-24	0	5	41	4	15	8	0	9	4	3	1
10-27 to 10-31	52	3	44	3	14	4	1	6	2	3	1
Activity totals (1)	2	27	193	22	61	27	3	32	16	19	6
× Activity factors (2)	0.15	0.3	0.5	0.25	0.4	0.15	0.15	0.25	0.15	0.4	0.25
= Total time per activity (hours) (3)	0.75	8.1	96.5	5.5	24.4	4.05	0.45	8.0	2.4	7.6	1.5

HRAs w/weight loss diagnosis (4)	HRAs w/inadequate intake diagnosis (5)	Total direct care time (6) 159.25 hours	Total paid time (7) 184 hours	Productivity factor (%) (8) 87%
No.: 152 / 79%	No.:156 / 81%			

Figure 5.2   Completed Direct Care Activity Individual Summary Form

Abbreviations: HR, high risk; HRA, high-risk assessment; MR, moderate risk.

Instructions:

Use weekly totals from the Direct Care Activity Tracking forms (Appendixes F.5 or F.6) to do the following:

1. List monthly totals for activities.
2. Insert activity factors.
3. Multiply each activity total by its activity factor.
4. List number of HRAs with nutrition diagnosis of weight loss, as well as percentage of total HRAs completed.
5. List number of HRAs with nutrition diagnosis of inadequate intake, as well as percentage of total HRAs completed.
6. Add time totals for each activity from "Total time per activity" row.
7. Obtain total paid time from payroll report or calculate.
8. Calculate productivity factor (%): (Total direct care time ÷ Total paid time) × 100.

Month __October__

Staff Names	Nutrition Screening	Nutrition Assessment: MR	Nutrition Assessment: High Risk (HRA)	Reassessment MR	Reassessment HR	Calorie Counts HR	Calorie Counts MR	Basic Education HR	Basic Education MR	Complex Education HR	Complex Education MR
CD	5	27	193	22	61	27	3	32	16	19	6
RA	2	30	179	19	65	14	2	24	9	16	4
JB	7	26	182	15	70	15	2	20	4	10	2
MD	4	10	195	2	90	5	1	10	2	2	1
Activity totals (1)	18	93	749	58	286	61	8	86	31	47	13
× Activity factors (2)	0.15	0.3	0.5	0.25	0.4	0.15	0.15	0.25	0.15	0.4	0.25
= Total time per activity (hours) (3)	2.7	27.9	374.5 A	14.5	114.4 B	91.5 C	1.2	21.5 D	4.65	18.8 E	3.25

Summary cells:

HRAs w/weight loss diagnosis (4)	HRAs w/inadequate intake diagnosis (5) No.: 625 83%	Total direct care time (6) 592.6 hours	Total paid time (7) 736 hours	Productivity factor (%) (8) 80.5%
Total UOS (9) 2,370	High-Risk DC time (10) 538.4 hours	High-Risk UOS (11) 2,154		

No.: 593
79%

Figure 5.3 Completed Direct Care Activity Summary Form

Abbreviations: DC, direct care; HR, high risk; HRA, high-risk assessment; MR, moderate risk; UOS, units of service.

Instructions:

Use weekly totals from the Direct Care Activity Individual Summary forms (Appendix F.7) to do the following:

1. List monthly totals for activities.
2. Insert activity factors.
3. Multiply each activity total by its activity factor.
4. List number of HRAs with nutrition diagnosis of weight loss, as well as percentage of total HRAs completed.
5. List number of HRAs with nutrition diagnosis of inadequate intake, as well as percentage of total HRAs completed.
6. Add time totals for each activity from "Total time per activity" row.
7. Obtain total paid time from payroll report or calculate.
8. Calculate productivity factor: (Total direct care time ÷ Total paid time) × 100.
9. Calculate total UOS: Total direct care time × 4. (1 UOS = 15 minutes; 4 UOS per hour.)
10. Calculate high-risk DC time: A + B + C + D + E.
11. Calculate high-risk UOS: High-risk DC time × 4.

RD SM   October 2004   1 UOS = 15 minutes

Diagnosis or Clinic	January	February	March	April	May	June	July	August	September	October	November	December
Initial Weight Management	175	169	192	170	165	160	155	160	175	150	140	130
Follow-up Weight Management	130	124	145	136	120	115	100	95	130	125	90	70
Initial Diabetes Mellitus	125	112	100	115	90	110	115	105	110	112	100	95
Follow-up Diabetes Mellitus	100	74	66	85	65	70	80	65	90	95	82	60
Initial HPL	50	60	42	40	30	25	28	32	55	65	40	25
Follow-up HPL	20	35	16	25	15	10	12	15	25	30	15	10
Other—initial	5	10	8	15	12	4	6	5	10	12	4	3
Other—follow-up	4	6	5	10	8	4	3	3	8	8	2	2
Total UOS	609	590	574	596	505	498	499	480	603	597	473	395
Charges ($)	15,000	15,225	14,350	14,900	12,625	12,450	12,475	12,000	15,075	14,925	11,825	9,875
									Total annual UOS	6,419	Total annual charges	$160,475

Figure 5.4 Completed Outpatient Direct Care Tracking Form

Abbreviation: HPL, hyperlipidemia; UOS, units of service.

Instructions:

1. List number of UOS by clinic site or diagnosis for a breakdown of the type of work performed/care provided.
2. Transfer monthly staff totals to Outpatient Direct Care Annual Summary Report (Appendix F.10).

RD Names	January UOS	January $	February UOS	February $	March UOS	March $	April UOS	April $	May UOS	May $	June UOS	June $	July UOS	July $	August UOS	August $	September UOS	September $	October UOS	October $	November UOS	November $	December UOS	December $
5M	609	15,225	590	14,750	574	14,350	596	14,900	505	12,625	498	12,450	499	12,475	480	12,000	603	15,075	597	14,925	473	11,825	395	9,875
AC	295	7,375	325	8,125	300	7,500	250	6,250	275	6,875	230	5,750	225	5,625	200	5,000	305	7,625	310	7,750	220	5,500	165	4,125
KB	290	7,250	300	7,500	285	7,125	275	6,875	245	6,125	210	5,250	215	5,375	185	4,875	285	7,125	290	7,250	200	5,000	170	4,250

	January	February	March	April	May	June	July	August	September	October	November	December
Total monthly UOS	1,194	1,215	1,159	1,121	1,025	938	939	865	1,193	1,197	893	730
Total monthly charges ($)	29,850	30,375	28,975	28,025	25,625	23,450	23,475	21,625	29,825	29,925	22,325	18,250
									Total annual UOS	12,469	Total annual charges	$311,725

Figure 5.5 Completed Outpatient Direct Care Annual Summary Report

Abbreviation: UOS, units of service.

Instructions:

List UOS and charges for each registered dietitian (RD) by month (monthly totals are tracked with Outpatient Direct Care Tracking Form found in Appendix F.9).

the issues in greater depth than the use of volume data alone can permit. The use of several types of volume data, comparison of actual admissions and outpatient visits with budgeted numbers, and consideration of other relevant factors allow managers to identify sources of underperformance and make midyear changes to achieve budget targets.

In the inpatient setting, it is important to emphasize that revenues are an indicator of staff productivity, not of the amount of money clinical nutrition services contribute to a facility's bottom line. The reason is because Medicare and most third party payers provide facilities a bundled payment for inpatient care based on patient diagnosis and bed type. In other words, charges for clinical nutrition services are not reimbursed directly. Therefore, implementing charges for new nutrition services and increasing the amount of charges for current services and products rarely generate more money for the facility.

The situation is different in the outpatient setting, in which direct reimbursement for medical nutrition therapy (MNT) is provided by Medicare and other third-party payers. To assess the contribution of outpatient clinical nutrition services to their organizations' bottom lines, managers often track collections, in addition to charges. Managers realize that the amount of charges collected may be considerably below the amounts billed, depending on facility procedures for collection. A comparison of revenues and collections with total activity volumes and costs for providing services allows managers to make an accurate evaluation of performance.

Expenses incurred for the care of Medicare inpatients, including registered dietitian's (RD's) time, are reported to the Centers for Medicare and Medicaid Services (CMS) on the facility's Medicare cost report. The amount of time reported to CMS for inpatient nutrition care by RDs who are hospital employees should reflect an accurate distribution of their workload between the inpatient and outpatient settings; in other words, only the actual time RDs spend in the inpatient setting should be listed on the Medicare cost report. Facilities cannot charge outpatients for Medicare Part B MNT provided by inpatient RDs whose total time has been reported on the Medicare cost report, because this method would appear to involve charging CMS twice for the same RD time. In-depth information on the topic of reimbursement is available from American Dietetic Association (ADA) publications and on-line resources.

Time Use

Another method used to measure productivity is the calculation of a productivity ratio that can be compared over time with a goal ratio. The ratio is created by comparing time spent performing direct care activities with either the total amount of time worked by staff or the total amount of time paid to staff. Paid time includes paid leave, whereas worked time does not.

Activity volumes for a specific interval (eg, a month) are obtained from manual reports or automated systems. The total number of each activity completed by all staff is multiplied by its predetermined *activity factor* (ie, the time allowed to complete the activity, with the term *allowed* referring to the fact that actual time spent on an activity may be longer or shorter than the activity factor). For productivity purposes, all staff members use a standard time for each activity. Determination of activity factors was described in detail in Chapter 3.

The total time spent on direct care activities by all clinical nutrition staff during the interval of data collection is determined by adding the individual staff members' activity time totals for all direct care activities. This figure is the numerator of the productivity ratio.

Occasionally, staff at a facility may work with a consultant who advises the use of a single activity factor for all activities performed; this factor is derived, with the consultant's assistance, from in-depth time studies conducted at the facility. In these cases, the total number of clinical nutrition activities is determined by adding the individual activity totals. This number is multiplied by the single activity factor to derive the total direct care time. This type of system was used by the author in a previous position. An activity factor of 0.3333 (⅓) of an hour was used for each activity, regardless of activity type.

The total amount of worked time for all staff members is obtained from payroll reports or from tracking forms used by staff members to record their activities. It is necessary to define a standard system for capturing time to ensure consistency and accuracy in the process. The total amount of time worked should be in the same unit used for total clinical activities (ie, minutes or hours). This number is the denominator of the productivity ratio. Box 5.1 illustrates an example of the calculation of a productivity ratio.

Managers may prefer to evaluate productivity using paid time instead of work time. If so, the amount of time used for the denominator is the total paid time for the staff involved in direct nutrition care. This number is used with the numerator of total amount of time spent for direct care activities.

Other types of data also can be used for the denominator in productivity ratios. Examples include patient days, adjusted patient days, adjusted occupied beds, and adjusted discharges. The decision to use different ratios is facility specific. Internal benchmarking can be done by comparing productivity ratios over a period of time. However, external benchmarking requires the use of the same ratios used as benchmark partners.

In the Premier external benchmarking program described in Chapter 3, numbers of direct care activities completed by dietitians are converted to workload units (WLUs) by multiplying the total number of each activity performed by the activity's WLU factor. This is the numerator for each of several productivity ratios (eg, WLU per worked hours, WLU per paid hours, WLU per patient day, and WLU per adjusted patient day). Use of the Premier program provides participating facilities with the opportunity for external benchmarking with other acute care facilities across the United States.

Box 5.1   Productivity Ratio: Determination of Numerator and Denominator

Numerator (choose 1)
- Number of activities
- Units of service (UOS)
- Hours worked in direct care activities (This is the sum of the number of individual direct care activities completed by staff members × the activity factors in hours for each direct care activity.)

Denominator (choose 1)
- Total hours worked
- Total hours paid
- Patient days
- Adjusted patient days (APD)
- Adjusted occupied beds
- Adjusted discharges

Examples
- Hours worked in direct care activities/Total hours paid
- UOS/APD
- Hours worked in direct care activities/APD

Productivity Factor or Percentage

Still another way to evaluate productivity is to convert time-based productivity ratios—that is, ratios in which the numerator and denominator are in the same units of time—to productivity factors or percentages. Box 5.2 and Table 5.1 show the formula for calculating a productivity factor and an example of a calculation.

Productivity factors for individual staff members and for the department as a whole can be compared with a target productivity factor. The target productivity factor will vary by facility, depending on the amount of indirect care and nonpatient care activities in which staff are involved. Staff should be included in determining targets to promote their acceptance of data collection and initiatives to evaluate and improve productivity. Performance improvement efforts should focus on increasing productivity over time from a baseline level. Improved productivity factors indicate success in these efforts. Productivity factors that reach a plateau below targets may indicate that maximum efficiencies have been reached and point to a need for larger systems changes to achieve any further improvements.

Any factors that reduce the total number of direct care nutrition activities performed will affect the productivity factors of individual staff members and of the department as a whole. For example, the productivity percentage of an RD who works in a critical care unit may be lower than that of an RD who works on a general medicine unit. As with activity volumes, emphasis should be placed on aggregate productivity

Box 5.2   Productivity Factor (Percentage)

Formula

$$\frac{\text{Numerator}}{\text{Denominator}} \times 100$$

Numerator

Total hours worked in direct care activities. This is the sum of the following (in hours):

- Number of nutrition screens × Activity factor
- Number of nutrition assessments × Activity factor
- Number of reassessments × Activity factor
- Number of calorie counts × Activity factor
- Number of basic nutrition education consults × Activity factor
- Number of complex nutrition education consults × Activity factor

Denominator (choose 1)

- Total hours worked
- Total hours paid

Examples

$$\frac{\text{Hours Worked in Direct Care Activities}}{\text{Total Hours Paid}} \times 100$$

$$\frac{\text{Hours Worked in Direct Care Activities}}{\text{Total Hours Worked}} \times 100$$

and assessment of overall department performance. In addition, sharing individual staff member productivity factors with the entire staff should be avoided. Individual data are more appropriately used for individual performance evaluation and goal setting.

The paid productivity factor will be influenced by both the benefits package at the facility and the number of long-term staff members, because these individuals usually have more paid time off than do staff members with shorter tenures of employment. For example, the paid productivity factor will be lower if all staff members have 3 weeks of vacation leave each year instead of 2 weeks. In a similar manner, assuming that senior staff accrue more paid leave, the paid productivity factor will be lower for a staff composed of individuals with long tenure, compared with a staff whose members have been employed fewer than 5 years.

Direct Care Time Distribution

Direct care activity time can be broken down further, if desired, to assess the distribution and appropriateness of staff time use. The pro-

Table 5.1   Example: Paid Productivity Factor

In this example, there are five full-time RDs. Activity factors have been predetermined via audit (column 2). Total number of activities completed in this example month by all five RDs are listed in column 3. Total calculated direct care times for each activity are listed in column 4.

Activity	Activity Factor (h)	Total No. of Activities Completed	Total Time (h)
Nutrition screening	0.25	500	125
Nutrition assessments—moderate risk	0.3	150	45
Nutrition assessments—high risk	0.5	250	125
Nutrition reassessments—moderate risk	0.2	75	15
Nutrition reassessments—high risk	0.4	550	220
Patient education	0.3	100	30
Calorie counts	0.25	50	12.5
		Total Time	**572.5**

$$\text{Productivity Factor (\%)} = \frac{\text{Total Direct Care Time}}{\text{Total Paid Time from Calculation or Payroll Reports}} \times 100$$

Calculation:

$$\frac{5\,\text{RDs} \times 2{,}080\,\text{h/y}}{12} = 867\,\text{h}$$

Productivity Factor = (572.5/867) × 100 = 66%

portion of time spent on specific activities can be determined by dividing the total time spent on the activity by the total time for all direct care activities and multiplying by 100:

$$\frac{\text{Amount of Time in Individual Activity}}{\text{Total Direct Care Time}} \times 100$$

Where: individual activities may include rescreening, nutrition assessment, reassessment, or patient education; and the amount of time in individual activity and total direct care time are measured with the same units (eg, hours or minutes).

If activity data indicate that 35% of staff time is spent in nutrition rescreening, 45% in nutrition assessment, and only 20% in monitoring and reassessment, performance improvement activities might focus on ways to streamline the rescreening process or on extending the number of days until rescreening is needed so that more time can be spent on monitoring and reassessment activities.

Job Satisfaction and Additional Human Resources Indicators

In evaluating department performance, managers often calculate and monitor human resources (HR) indicators that affect productivity; examples include annual turnover rate, controllable turnover rate, vacancy rate, average days of absenteeism per full-time equivalent per year, and average length of staff tenure. From a JCAHO perspective, it is important that the definition of these terms and their methods of calculation be consistent with definitions and methods adopted by the facility, to promote accurate use of indicators in facility-wide staffing effectiveness initiatives (2). Sample definitions are shown in Box 5.3.

Another HR indicator that managers can monitor is the job satisfaction of clinical nutrition staff. The importance of job satisfaction was indicated by its inclusion on the JCAHO list of HR indicators. Many facilities conduct formal assessments of staffing satisfaction at regular intervals—for example, every 2 to 3 years—using available survey tools like the Gallup poll. The usefulness of these data in assessing clinical nutrition staff satisfaction depends on the ability to subdivide the department data into subsets of staff (to derive the data for the clinical nutrition staff). When available, information derived from staff satisfaction surveys can provide insight into problems that are identified through the use of other HR indicators, such as turnover rate or absenteeism.

Another tool used to assess job satisfaction is the Job Descriptive Index (JDI), developed by Smith and colleagues (3). The original JDI measures five facets of job satisfaction: work on present job, present

---

Box 5.3   Sample Definitions

1. Patient Satisfaction With Nutrition Services
Patient opinion of the nutrition services received during the hospital stay as determined by scaled responses to a uniform set of questions designed to elicit patient views on aspects of service, administered to a sample of all patients admitted to the hospital for acute care.

2. Staff Vacancy Rate
The number of open positions per quarter divided by the total number of positions per quarter multiplied by 100.

3. Overtime Rate
The number of hours worked beyond 40 hours a week (overtime) by hourly regular employees per month divided by the number of regular staff worked hours per month multiplied by 100.

pay, opportunities for promotion, supervision, and coworkers. A sixth scale, the Job in General scale, has been added to the original version of the JDI (4). Use of a tool such as the JDI provides comparative data with existing norms, allows identification of specific strengths and weaknesses within a work group, and facilitates monitoring of changes in these factors over time. Recognition of strengths can build morale, whereas recognition of weaknesses points to areas where improvements can be made.

The full six-scale JDI contains 90 items. An abridged version contains 25 items. The JDI has been validated, has standards for normative comparisons, and is available for purchase.

Studies of job satisfaction of dietitians have been reported in the literature. Findings from past studies using the JDI consistently showed that dietitian satisfaction was lowest with pay and opportunities for promotion and highest with the level of supervision provided. Researchers noted that when compared with norms, dietitians were more likely to have lower satisfaction with pay and promotion opportunities than individuals in positions requiring similar levels of education and training (5,6).

In a 2002 study, researchers used a different assessment tool, the Index of Job Satisfaction, to evaluate the job satisfaction of RDs (7). They noted higher job satisfaction when comparing survey results with normative data, along with positive associations between job satisfaction and both professional involvement and earning more than $60,000 per year. The results of this study need to be interpreted in the context of the demographics of the respondents to the survey. More than 85% of the responding RDs were older than 44 years, whereas 53.4% of ADA membership is older than 41 years.

Data from the 1999 update of the ADA membership database provide information on salaries of dietitians and dietetic technicians (8). Although salaries have improved over the years and the levels of salary increase are consistent with levels for other health care professionals, salary continues to be an issue for many individuals within the dietetics profession.

Evaluation of Nutrition Care and Services

Department managers and staff can expand their evaluation of the volume of nutrition care provided by determining how well the established time standards for completion of nutrition interventions are met. They can also evaluate the impact of their care and activities on customer perceptions of the service received.

Process Monitoring

Data on completion of nutrition care activities and adherence to established time standards can be converted to service indicators that can be tracked over time. Although other types of performance data could be collected, compliance with JCAHO standards affects the quality of patient care, facility accreditation status, and, potentially, patient safety. As a result, these data and their corresponding indicators are more likely to be important to upper-level facility managers and administrators. Examples of these service indicators include the following:

- Nutrition screening
  - ➤ Completion within 24 hours of admission (See Appendix F.11 for form.)
  - ➤ Referral of at-risk patients to dietitians for follow-up evaluation (See Appendix F.11 for form.)
- Nutrition assessment
  - ➤ Completion according to time standard or standards defined in policy (See Appendix F.12 for form.)
  - ➤ Definition of specific, measurable, timed goals in plan of care (See Appendix F.12 for form.)
  - ➤ Physician adherence to dietitian recommendations
  - ➤ Time elapsed from dietitian recommendations to writing of physician orders and implementation of recommendations
- Monitoring and reassessment
  - ➤ Completion according to time standard or standards defined in policy or nutrition care plan (See Appendix F.13 for form.)
  - ➤ Documentation of status of nutrition problems and achievement of goals (See Appendix F.13 for form.)
  - ➤ Completion of discharge planning

Inpatient Patient Satisfaction

JCAHO has indicated the importance of patient satisfaction by including both patient complaints and family complaints on its list of approved clinical/service indicators. Managers should determine if their facilities have selected one or both of these indicators for monitoring. When possible, managers and clinical nutrition staff will want to be included in facility-wide activities and unit-specific initiatives to evaluate patient satisfaction. However, even managers who are not included in facility-wide initiatives can obtain facility patient and family satisfaction and complaint data and conduct their own analyses, in order to identify associations between performance levels of these service indicators and the HR indicators being tracked. Care must be used in assigning accountability for scores, whether low or high, entirely to the performance of the clinical nutrition staff, because many variables affect patient satisfaction.

Outpatient Customer Satisfaction

In the outpatient setting, measuring customer satisfaction and meeting or exceeding customer expectations for service are increasingly important; reasons include changing patterns of reimbursement and increasing patient out-of-pocket payments for health care. Most facilities with outpatient programs conduct customer satisfaction evaluations to assess performance. Nutrition managers can use these data in their own evaluation initiatives, although at some facilities, large time delays occur between customer appointments and distribution of customer satisfaction data. This delay may make it difficult to identify retrospectively the factors that affected the available scores. In addition, the overall number of MNT patients who complete customer satisfaction surveys may be small, limiting the validity of results.

As an alternative, outpatient nutrition clinics may choose to provide customers with short evaluation forms that can be completed and mailed in with the feedback needed. Other methods include telephone surveys and questionnaires completed on-site. Any evaluation process should encourage accurate responses and ensure client anonymity in order to gather valuable information but not create anxiety about the impact of responses on care. A method that allows written feedback may be useful, because patients may hesitate to share direct verbal feedback. It may also be useful to request feedback only after clients have completed all planned MNT sessions.

A service indicator commonly used in the outpatient setting that can be used by outpatient nutrition clinics is the length of time to third available appointment—that is, the length of time a client would have to wait on the day of measurement if he or she called for an appointment, either an initial appointment or an appointment for follow-up. The reason for selecting the third available appointment as the point of evaluation is that it better reflects how long most patients have to wait for appointments. Last-minute cancellations can create the impression of appointment availability that few patients are able to take advantage of. A defined process for data collection is needed, and it must specify the measurement date (eg, the first business day of the month), type of appointment (eg, initial or follow-up), time of day of appointments, and frequency of monitoring.

A standard for time to the third available appointment does not exist for MNT appointments, although facility standards may exist (eg, within 2 weeks of contact). It is also reasonable to assume that the wait should be short enough to allow for the provision of MNT at the intervals defined in the *American Dietetic Association Medical Nutrition Therapy Evidence-Based Guides for Practice* (9). As an example, the initial MNT session for a woman with a new diagnosis of gestational diabetes mellitus would be scheduled within 1 week of physician referral, as defined in the MNT Guide for this diagnosis.

Long intervals between appointments are not conducive to effective monitoring of client progress and indicate the need for an assessment of the adequacy of appointment availability. It is important to evaluate the total number of appointments available and the time of day of appointment availability. For example, if the length of time until the next early evening appointment is 1 month, it may indicate a need to add more early evening appointment slots.

Outpatient nutrition clinics also can track other types of service indicators that matter to clients, such as the average length of waiting time from arrival for appointments to the beginning of MNT sessions.

Clinics can track their no-show rates (ie, the number of appointments that are kept by clients divided by the number of scheduled appointments multiplied by 100). High no-show rates can indicate many things, including a need for an appointment reminder system; excessive waiting times for appointments, which may spur clients to go to other providers or forgo MNT altogether; or insurance limitations on the number of covered MNT sessions that patients discovered after their initial sessions.

STAFFING EFFECTIVENESS

JCAHO requires facilities to evaluate their staffing effectiveness and has provided resources that managers and clinical nutrition staff can use in these efforts. Staffing effectiveness evaluations are to be completed at the facility level; however, they involve those departments whose levels of staffing directly or indirectly affect the HR and clinical/service indicators selected by the facility for data collection and monitoring. Although individual nutrition departments are not required to monitor staffing effectiveness separately from facility initiatives, in most hospitals, planning for staffing and collection of staffing data occur at the department or unit level.

Balanced Scorecard Approach

JCAHO promotes the use of a balanced scorecard approach to staffing effectiveness evaluation. Using this approach, clinical, service, and HR indicators are evaluated together to promote a better understanding of the relationships between data sets and to facilitate more effective problem solving. This approach involves collecting and reporting data for the same time interval—for example, monthly indicators for both high-risk nutrition assessments completed within the time standard and RD worked hours per adjusted patient day. Indicator data are easily displayed in a matrix and on a multiple-line graph. Refer to Table 5.2 for definitions of these performance indicator (PI) tools (10). In the example given, monitoring both HR indicators (RD worked hours per adjusted patient day) and service indicators (high-risk nutrition assessments completed within the time standard) over time and evaluating the impact of trends in the HR indicator on the service indicator allow associations to be made between levels of staffing and the ability to comply with JCAHO nutrition standards.

The methods described in this section are important ones to use in assessing the implementation of the staffing plan and productivity. They also allow departments to create HR and service indicators that can be used to evaluate their performance over time, compare their performance with benchmark partners who are tracking the same indicators, and compare their performance with best-practice reports in the literature, to the extent that they exist. In other words, these methods focus on what work is done and how much is accomplished. However, these indicators do not provide a way to demonstrate the

---

Balanced Scorecard Approach to Evaluating Staffing Effectiveness

To get a broad view of performance, several types of indicators should be tracked over time and be evaluated together:

- Human resources indicators
- Service indicators
- Clinical indicators

Table 5.2   Data Analysis Techniques

Technique	Description
Matrix	A table that displays combinations of numbers together over time (eg, indicator rates by month).
Multiple-line graph	A way to display matrix data. Lines for two to four indicators are graphed together.
	Graphing allows observation of relationships between indicator data and identification of time periods of lowest and highest performance of indicators, individually and in combination.
Spider diagram	A pictorial method of displaying data for a single period (eg, 1 month). Also known as a *radar chart*.
	Data for actual and average performance of each indicator are plotted as points on scales with ratings from 0 to ideal. Each scale forms a leg or spoke that radiates from a central point.
	Data points closest to the center of the circle are the lowest level of performance for the period measured.
Scatter diagram	A graph that shows how one variable relates to another. The diagram is intended to show the existence or lack of a relationship, not cause and effect.
	Multiple data points (preferably at least 30) must be plotted. The strength of a relationship can be determined by the pattern of the data points.
Pearson correlation	A table showing the correlation coefficients for the data listed in a matrix.
	Calculations can be performed using spreadsheets with this capability.
	The scale of coefficients ranges from −1 to +1.
	0 = no correlation.
	−1 = very strong negative correlation (eg, one indicator increases, one decreases).
	+1 = very strong positive relationship (eg, both indicators increase or decrease at the same time).
	−0.80 = moderate negative relationship.
	+0.80 = moderate positive relationship.

Source: Data are from reference 10.

impact of clinical nutrition staff and MNT on positive patient outcomes. What is really needed is a third set of indicators—clinical nutrition indicators—that can be used with the HR and service indicators to identify the impact of staffing levels on the quality of patient care provided.

For some managers and dietitians, the challenge of demonstrating the impact of MNT on patient outcomes in the acute care setting seems too complex to attempt, given the short lengths of stay of many inpatients and the interrelationships in the provision of health care. These interrelationships make it difficult to determine which types of care and team members produce outcomes and the extent of influence of many different variables.

Regardless of the challenges, managers have realized that without such systems, it will be increasingly difficult to demonstrate the need for clinical nutrition staff in the coming years. And although reductions in staffing already have been experienced in many facilities, they provide no protection against further reductions.

As with any large task, it is important to maintain a focus on the desired goal, start with small steps, and move incrementally toward the goal. It is also important to remember that at least initially, it is not necessary to demonstrate cause and effect between low levels of clinical nutrition staffing and poor patient outcomes. It is enough to begin by demonstrating associations or correlations between staffing and outcomes, especially outcomes valued by administrators and payers. This demonstration can be accomplished by tracking clinical indicators, in addition to HR and service indicators, and by conducting well-designed outcomes projects.

Linking Clinical Staffing With Patient Outcomes and Care

As noted, it is challenging for managers and clinical nutrition staff in the inpatient setting to establish a link between the outcomes of MNT and their HR indicators. Making this connection necessitates two things. First, it is necessary to demonstrate that a variation in the amount of MNT that patients receive produces a variation in outcomes. (Figure 5.6 illustrates the relationship between MNT for patients with nutrition problems and positive patient outcomes.) An outcomes project has this goal. Second, it must be shown that variations in staffing can be linked to variations in the amount of MNT that patients receive and the outcomes achieved. (Figure 5.7 illustrates how clinical nutrition staffing can affect the provision of MNT and result in positive patient outcomes.)

Types of Outcomes

Outcomes are the result or results of an intervention or the lack of an intervention. Outcomes are measured by determining change, or

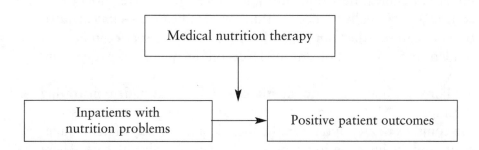

Figure 5.6 Contribution of MNT interventions to positive patient outcomes.

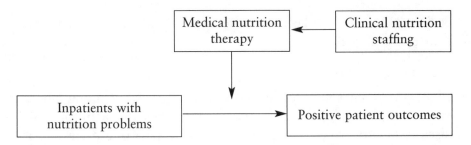

Figure 5.7 Effect of clinical nutrition staffing on MNT and positive patient outcomes.

sometimes lack of change, over time in an outcome indicator (ie, a piece of data that can be measured consistently and accurately and that is affected by the intervention being evaluated).

Time Frames

Outcomes occur in different time frames after an intervention, depending on the type of intervention and the nature of the problem for which an intervention is used. Time frames can be short term (ie, within a few hours or days), intermediate (ie, within a few weeks), or long term (ie, within months to years).

An example of a short-term outcome in the inpatient setting is the increase in energy, protein, vitamin, and mineral intake resulting from the provision of liquid nutritional supplements to inpatients with pressure ulcers via a medication pass program. An intermediate outcome is initial wound healing achieved on the subacute unit with continued use of the medication pass form of nutrition supplementation and monitoring of intake. Positive outcomes might be demonstrated by comparing improvements in wound stage with intake of energy, protein, and other nutrients.

Examples of long-term outcomes are completion of the wound-healing process, increased ability to perform activities of daily living, and decreased hospital readmissions, demonstrated by ongoing monitoring of weight, intake, and wound stage while continuing the medication pass program in the long-term care setting.

An example of a short-term outcome in the outpatient setting is a reduction in patient intake of saturated fat after an outpatient MNT session, determined by analyzing 24-hour recall data from initial and follow-up MNT sessions. An example of an intermediate outcome is the resulting reduction in total and low-density lipoprotein cholesterol observed at 6 weeks and 3 months after initiating MNT. A long-term outcome of MNT is the reduction in the incidence of new cardiac events over a 10-year period in a group of patients with hyperlipidemia who received MNT.

It is not surprising that data collection is harder and more involved the longer the time frame between the intervention and the measurement of the outcomes of interest. For this reason, most outcomes

projects focus on the collection and analysis of short-term and intermediate outcomes data.

Outcome Categories

Clinical outcomes may be divided into categories, including laboratory data, physical measurements, and the signs and symptoms of a
disease. Functional outcomes measure the impact of a disease or its
treatment on patients and clients; examples include the ability to perform activities of daily living, the ability to fulfill social and family
roles, and health-related quality of life. Behavioral outcomes, also
known as *therapeutic lifestyle outcomes,* are measures of the changes
that take place in illness- or treatment-related behaviors as a result of
intervention; examples are changes in eating-related behaviors such as
reading food labels, methods of food preparation, and food intake.
Economic outcomes measure the financial impact of an intervention.
Rates of disease incidence or prevalence are also measured.

To demonstrate the impact of MNT, managers must establish a
link between the more easily measured short-term patient outcomes
and intermediate or long-term outcomes, especially ones that have
health and financial implications. Because extended outcomes studies
are not generally feasible, this link can be achieved by conducting a
structured review of the literature to answer a clinical question that
links the short-term and intermediate and long-term outcomes.

In truth, the task of demonstrating the impact of inpatient MNT
on intermediate and long-term outcomes is a very formidable one.
This demonstration may well require multisite research conducted
through a practice-based research network, such as ADA's Dietetic
Practice—Based Research Network, to achieve success at the level
needed.

Core Measures for Evaluating Staffing Effectiveness

The evaluation of staffing effectiveness allows identification of associations between staffing, skill mix, competencies, and problems affecting patient care and safety, so that corrective actions can be taken. This
evaluation is another part of the "check" stage of the plan-do-check-
act continuous quality improvement cycle. As with the other stages of
the PI cycle, evaluation activities are most effective when performed by
a team composed of staff representing the areas involved in the
processes being evaluated.

Checking involves comparing data and indicators of actual performance (HR, service, and clinical) with desired levels of performance. Desired levels of performance are obtained from strategic plans,
budget goals, performance in prior years, and external benchmarks.

It is important to evaluate selected HR, service, and clinical indicator data individually, identifying trends in data over time. However,
the most useful information is obtained by evaluating the indicators in
combination, using appropriate data correlation and analysis tech-

niques (ie, the balanced scorecard approach). In fact, issues related to skill mix and competency are more likely to become apparent at this level of data analysis.

Because it is cumbersome and costly to track a large number of indicators, managers will want to select a set of core measures that can be used to measure performance rather than tracking all possible indicators. Ideally, these core measures can be incorporated into facility-wide staffing effectiveness initiatives. See Appendix F.21 for a form to use in selecting indicators.

Ideally, three types of data or performance indicators are used for this type of evaluation: HR, service, and clinical. Examples of indicators to track for this purpose in the inpatient setting include the following:

- HR indicators
  - ➤ Percentage of days in compliance with the staffing plan*
  - ➤ RD (or RD and dietetic technician, registered [DTR]) paid hours per adjusted patient days*
  - ➤ RD (or RD and DTR) worked hours per adjusted patient days
  - ➤ Clinical nutrition staff vacancy rate
- Service indicators
  - ➤ Number of direct care activities, units of service (UOS), or WLUs per adjusted occupied beds or adjusted patient days—all patients or high-risk patients only*
  - ➤ Amount of direct nutrition care time per adjusted occupied beds or adjusted patient days—all patients or high-risk patients only*
  - ➤ Percentage compliance with time standard for high-risk nutrition assessment
  - ➤ Percentage compliance with time standard for high-risk nutrition monitoring/reassessment
- Clinical indicators—Clinical indicators for nutrition care and MNT have not been well defined. This list presents options for consideration.
  - ➤ Percentage change between number of high-risk patients with nutrition diagnosis of weight loss at initial assessment and reassessment*
  - ➤ Percentage change between number of high-risk patients with nutrition diagnosis of inadequate intake at initial assessment and reassessment*
  - ➤ Percentage achievement of nutrition care plan goals for high-nutrition-risk patients at initial assessment and reassessment
  - ➤ Percentage achievement of nutrient (eg, energy and protein) requirements for high-nutrition-risk patients at initial assessment and reassessment
  - ➤ Indicator data and rates compiled from minimum data set (MDS) forms (subacute units)

The indicators with an asterisk (*) have been selected for inclusion in a potential set of core measures. However, managers can define their own sets of core measures using these indicators or others of their own choosing. Ideally, managers will begin to use sets of core measure that include all three types of indicators and will report their use in the literature; this reporting may lead to eventual consensus on a set of core measures within the profession.

Appendixes F.14, F.15, and F.16 contain forms for tracking indicator data by type of indicator (ie, HR, service, and clinical). Appendix F.17 contains a form to use in summarizing performance on the core measures, the "Staffing Effectiveness Indicator Matrix." Forms for measuring clinical effectiveness and calculating the clinical indicators marked with an asterisk (*) can be found in Appendixes F.18, F.19, and F.20.

Managers and staff will need to evaluate current systems of documentation and methods for collecting performance improvement audit data to ensure that the data needed for calculation of clinical indicator rates are collected. As with any data collection process, procedures should allow calculation of indicators despite occasional missing or incomplete data. Missing data, although undesirable, occur for a variety of reasons in day-to-day practice. Some data can be retrieved when omissions are identified, but this retrieval is not always possible.

Performance Improvement

The magnitude and causes of problems should be investigated using PI tools such as fishbone diagrams, histograms, and Pareto charts. JCAHO has published a useful resource for this work: *Tools for Performance Measurement in Health Care: A Quick Reference Guide* (11). Priorities for correction of problems should be determined to ensure that team time is used effectively and focused on issues most likely to show positive results.

Implementation of solutions and strategies occurs at the "act" stage of the continuous quality improvement cycle. As when implementing any procedure or project, it is important to have specific information in the implementation plan, including information on action steps to be taken, information on accountability for accomplishing tasks, and a timeline for completion of tasks. The implementation plan needs to incorporate steps to monitor the effectiveness of strategies used to correct targeted problems. PI strategies should lead to improvements in the HR, service, and clinical indicators collected over time.

Once data indicate that targeted problems have been corrected, facilities may identify additional data to track, leading to the identification of new performance issues. With new PI initiatives, the continuous quality improvement cycle of plan-do-check-act begins again.

Planning an Outcomes Project

As discussed previously, demonstrating the impact of MNT in the inpatient setting is challenging. Short lengths of hospital stay and the collaborative nature of health care are factors. So is the tendency for dietitians to view research and projects that include data collection as beyond their area of expertise or interest, although some facilities now include the use of current research in their annual performance appraisal and competency assessment processes. With careful thought and planning and a set of tools for collecting outcomes data, managers and clinical nutrition staff can lay a firm foundation for their outcomes work.

Initial outcomes projects need not be sophisticated. Small projects give staff opportunities to learn firsthand about practice-based research and to expand their research knowledge and skills. Questions that invariably arise during projects lead staff to answers that can be applied to future projects. Sharing new information and the results of projects may lead to additional feedback and enhanced recognition for MNT and the RDs. And important links can be established between the ability to achieve outcomes and levels of clinical nutrition staffing.

The goal of an outcomes project is to demonstrate the impact of MNT on patient outcomes. This section describes the steps in an outcomes project, and Appendix F.22 contains a worksheet for conducting an outcomes project.

Step 1: Define a Practice Question

The first step in planning an outcomes project is to define a practice question that is of interest to staff and is relevant to department and facility goals. As an example, the return of a large amount of unopened tube-feeding products to the central kitchen over a period of time might prompt dietitians to ask if patients receiving tube feedings are meeting their nutritional requirements and receiving the ordered amounts of tube feedings. In this example, department goals could be achieved by reducing the labor costs associated with collecting unused tube-feeding products and returning them to the central kitchen. Also, department goals could be met by reducing the supply costs associated with maintaining an excess inventory of tube-feeding products on the patient care units and in the central kitchen.

The following are other examples of practice questions:

- Does our nutrition screening process identify patients at nutritional risk?
- Are patients meeting the goals defined in their nutrition care plans?
- Do physicians follow the recommendations made by the dietitians for the type and amount of patients' nutrition support?
- Following discharge, do patients remember and use the survival skills nutrition information they receive in the hospital?

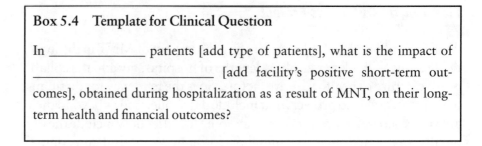

- Following discharge, do patients with weight loss continue the improvements in weight status started in the hospital?
- Do patients referred for postdischarge MNT follow-up counseling receive it?

Practice questions are refined into what are known as *clinical questions*. Each clinical question includes four parts: a patient population or group, an intervention, a comparison group or treatment, and an outcome to be measured. Clinical questions are sometimes referred to as *PICO questions,* using an acronym created from the first letters of the four parts of the question (population, intervention, comparison group, and outcome). (Box 5.4 provides a template to use in writing a clinical question.)

Step 2: Review the Literature

The second step in planning an outcomes project is a review of the professional literature relevant to the clinical question. A literature review provides background for the project and helps define types of outcomes to collect and methods of data collection. It also can let staff know if others have had the same or a similar clinical question and, if so, the results that have been reported. Staff members should use a structured process for conducting their literature reviews to ensure soundness of methods and accessing of existing literature reviews and patient care guidelines that are relevant to their clinical questions. One recommended approach to literature review, the 4S (systems, synopses, syntheses, and studies) approach, is described in Table 5.3 (12,13).

The 4S approach begins with a search for systematic literature reviews and summaries, known as *evidence analyses,* that have been completed by other clinicians. These systems, synopses, and syntheses are the first three of the four Ss.

When no systematic reviews or abstracts are found or when time has elapsed since their reporting, staff members need to search the literature for studies, the fourth S, by initiating a PubMed query. The ADA Web site contains a link to the National Library of Medicine PubMed Web site for quick access and instructions on the process.

Prior to initiating a query, staff members should define criteria for their literature search, including the types of articles to be reviewed, the time frame for article publication, language, and subject type. They should note the following suggestions for search criteria:

Table 5.3   4S Approach to Literature Review

Information Source	Definition	Examples
Systems	Information sources that cover a variety of diagnoses, provide a summary of the results of high-quality systematic reviews, and are updated frequently	• *Clinical Evidence* (http://www.clinicalevidence.com) • *American Dietetic Association Medical Nutrition Therapy Evidence-Based Guides for Practice* [CD-ROMs] • National Guideline Clearing-house Web site (http://www.guidelines.gov)
Synopses	Structured abstracts of high-quality systematic reviews or original articles	• American College of Physicians (ACP) Journal Club (http://www.acpjc.org) • Evidence-Based Medicine (http://ebm.bmjjournals.com) • National Guideline Clearing-house Web site (http://www.guidelines.gov)
Syntheses	High-quality systematic review articles	• Cochrane Database of Systematic Reviews (http://www.update-software.com/Cochrane) • Database of Abstracts of Reviews of Effectiveness (http://agatha.york.ac.uk/darehp.htm)
Studies	Primary research specific to the type of clinical question being asked	• Journal articles obtained by search of one or more data-bases (eg, MEDLINE)

Source: Data are from references 12 and 13.

- *Type of article.* First choice: randomized controlled trials or clinical controlled studies; also acceptable: nonrandomized trials, observational studies, and cohort or case control studies
- *Population.* Humans with an age range similar to the patient population being studied in the outcomes project
- *Sample size.* At least 10 patients for each intervention or group studied
- *Setting.* Similar to the setting being studied in the outcomes project
- *Time frame for publication.* Within the last 5 years
- *Language.* English

A search often produces a long list of articles, some of which may not be relevant to the clinical question. Staff members should scan the list of article titles and eliminate the articles that do not meet the search criteria selected. For example, a title indicating animal research would be eliminated, as would an article on research in long-term care when the clinical question is specific to adult patients in the acute care setting. Once this step has been completed, staff members should read the abstracts of the articles that remain and eliminate additional articles that are not relevant. The third level of review—the review of entire articles—should be completed for the articles that remain on the list after title scanning and abstract review.

In recent years, there has been much discussion about the importance of evaluating the quality of evidence in individual articles or studies, because publication in a peer-reviewed journal does not automatically signal a high level of evidence quality. ADA has adopted a method of evidence analysis, based on the Institute for Clinical Systems Improvement (ICSI) method, that dietitians can use to review a single article or a set of articles obtained through a literature search (14). According to the ICSI-based method, information from each article is summarized on a worksheet. Next, each article is rated using a quality ratings score sheet. One of three ratings or quality scores is given, based on the answers to the questions listed on the score sheet: a plus sign (+) for positive, a minus sign (–) for negative, or a zero (0) for neutral. A list is made of all articles reviewed and their evidence quality scores.

The literature review concludes by determining an answer to the original clinical question, stated in the form of a recommendation for patient care. The recommendation should be based on the results of the article reviews and their quality scores. Once defined, the recommendation is given a grade, ranging from grade I to grade IV, indicating the strength of the available evidence to support the recommendation. The recommendation that is formulated defines the intervention to be tested in the outcomes project.

Step 3: Specify Study Design

The next step in planning an outcomes project is to specify the study design. The characteristics of the population to be studied must be defined—that is, which patients are included and which patients are not included. These characteristics, listed in the project's inclusion and exclusion criteria, should define any exclusions for comorbid conditions or diseases. Because of time limitations, it may be necessary to collect data from a sample or portion of the population that meets the project's criteria.

A statistician can assist in determining the sample size needed to demonstrate an effect of MNT. Some facilities have statisticians on staff. Others have staff in their PI departments who can assist with this step of project planning. Nearby university nutrition departments are another resource, as are colleagues who are experienced with research methods. If a statistician is not available, a reasonable number of patients to include in a sample is 25 to 30.

The sampling method should ensure that the sample selected accurately represents the entire group of patients defined in the inclusion and exclusion criteria, in order to allow generalization of the results of the project to the entire group. Sampling can be accomplished by randomly choosing patients who meet the inclusion and exclusion criteria or by limiting data collection to a defined time period, assuming that the period selected accurately reflects usual conditions.

Step 4: Define Study Methods

The next step in planning an outcomes projects is to define the study methods. Whenever possible, the project should include a control or comparison group. Outcome indicators or types of data should be selected and defined, and data collection methods must be specified. With the many limitations on time, it may be necessary to limit types of data to those items collected in routine practice and to use existing forms as data collection forms. However, despite time limitations, it is important to collect data that could affect the results of the project (eg, changes in medications and new diagnoses or relevant comorbidities).

Consistency in study methods, including methods used to assess appetite and nutrient intake, is very important. As an example, appetite can be assessed consistently by having patients record their level of appetite on an appetite analogue scale ranging from 1 to 10 prior to each meal or for the prior 24-hour period. Patients assessing intake for the prior 24 hours might indicate the lowest level of appetite experienced during the past 24 hours. If intake of supplements is being evaluated, a method of recording consumption needs to be defined (eg, providing patients with a log for recording daily consumption in ounces or quarter-can increments).

Study methods should include a process for checking data at regular intervals to ensure that missing data can be collected while patients and their medical records are still available. Study methods should be spelled out clearly and put into a format that can be used to train staff.

Plans should include a small pilot study to test project procedures and forms. Pilot studies can save valuable staff time by allowing needed changes to be identified and revisions to be made before a large number of patients are involved. It may be necessary to obtain approval of the facility's institutional review board (IRB) or a waiver from IRB review, depending on the type of project and the plans for sharing data and results after project completion. Recent changes in the laws related to sharing patient data, even what is known as "de-identified data," make adherence to IRB procedures very important. The process can be initiated by contacting a member of the IRB for information and assistance. Managers and clinical nutrition staff will find that working with an IRB provides an excellent opportunity for learning about research.

Step 5: Determine How Project Data Will Be Analyzed

The next step in the planning process is to determine how the project data will be analyzed. Ideally, this step takes place in two parts: early in the planning process and prior to beginning the project. Early in planning, it is helpful to meet with a statistician to discuss the clinical question, data collection, and data aggregation and analysis. Prior to project implementation, it is helpful to review final plans for data analysis with the statistician to ensure that all questions have been answered. Once data have been collected, the statistician can be very helpful in data analysis and interpretation of results. RDs without access to a statistician can generate descriptive summaries and perform simple calculations (eg, means, medians, ranges, and correlation coefficients). User-friendly computer software packages for data analysis are helpful.

Step 6: Define the Timeline

The final step in the planning process is to define a timeline for the project. It is important to be realistic in developing the timeline, allowing adequate time for the project to be completed while keeping the timeline to a manageable length. Projects that extend too long may not reach completion.

The methods just described can be used in both the inpatient and outpatient settings. They make up the ideal approach to planning an outcomes project. However, time limitations and the need to introduce outcomes data collection to staff in small segments may dictate that study design and data collection methods be simplified. As staff members gain experience and confidence in conducting outcomes research, the complexity of projects can be increased.

Application in the Inpatient Setting

Designing Outcomes Projects

Managers and dietitians can enhance the likelihood of a successful outcomes project in the inpatient setting by limiting the scope of initial projects to the collection of short-term outcomes data. It is also helpful to focus on high-risk patients and outcome indicators that are affected by MNT and nutrition care (eg, nutrient intake, percentage of nutrient requirements met, weight change, and achievement of goals defined in the nutrition care plan).

As staff members gain more experience, they can expand the scope of their outcomes projects to assessment of the impact of inpatient MNT on intermediate outcomes (outcomes observed in the days and weeks after discharge from the hospital). The identification of positive associations provides support for the importance of inpatient RDs and the MNT they provide. Examples of outcome indicators that might be assessed after discharge include nutrient intake, percentage of nutrient requirements met, tolerance of nutrition support, understanding and use of nutrition guidelines, and weight.

As noted earlier, projects should include a control or comparison group. Initially this inclusion may seem to add an unacceptable level of complexity to a project. However, depending on the type of project, patients may be able to serve as their own controls through measurement of outcomes before and after initiation of an intervention in the same patients. Alternatively, the same outcomes can be measured in two groups of similar inpatients—in one group of patients before the implementation of an intervention, such as an MNT guide or a new nutrition assessment procedure, and in a second group of patients after implementation. An example of an outcomes project can be found in Box 5.5.

Inpatient MNT Protocols

In response to third party payer demand, MNT protocols have been developed by groups of volunteer ADA members in conjunction with ADA staff and the Quality Management Committee. Until recently, the focus of the volunteer groups was on protocol development for the outpatient and private practice settings. As a result, ADA guides or protocols for MNT in the inpatient setting are not yet available. Thus, dietitians practicing in this setting have not had the opportunities

---

Box 5.5   Outcomes Project Example

Clinical Question

Does implementation of an enteral nutrition support (ENS) care protocol result in improved patient outcomes compared with the outcomes of patients who did not receive ENS according to the care protocol?

Population

50 inpatients on enteral nutrition support (25 in the comparison group and 25 in the intervention group):
Comparison group: 25 patients studied immediately prior to ENS protocol implementation
Intervention group: 25 patients studied immediately after implementation of the protocol

Intervention

Enteral nutrition support care protocol

Data Collection—Intervention

- Monitoring key protocol interventions to ensure that implementation occurred and to check for interventions in the comparison group without use of care protocol (ie, Were interventions completed even though they were not part of the actual care protocol?)
- Initiating ENS per protocol
- Ordering laboratory tests per protocol and reviewing results
- Daily monitoring of amount of ENS ordered and amount actually infused
- Communicating with the MD when variances are identified; recommending change in type and/or amount of ENS

Data Collection—Outcomes

- Improvement in body weight (nonfluid)
- Tolerance of tube feeding—absence of nausea, vomiting, diarrhea, high residuals, and/or electrolyte imbalances
- Percentage of nutrient requirements met (energy and protein)
- Percentage of ordered tube feeding administered: (Delivered amount/Ordered amount) × 100

available to practitioners in the outpatient and private practice settings to gain experience using MNT protocols to guide MNT provision and the collection of individual and aggregate outcomes data.

ADA protocols for inpatient MNT also could be used effectively in the acute care setting, where the use of clinical paths and care maps is well established. Certainly, the use of such protocols would promote consistent patient care and provide a tool to define staffing needs and evaluate staffing effectiveness.

Dietitians employed in nutrition departments at hospitals that have contracted with various management services have access to a set of inpatient protocols developed specifically for their accounts. Other facilities have developed their own MNT protocols. For example, at Vanderbilt University Medical Center, MNT protocols for both adult and pediatric inpatients are used to guide the provision of nutrition care for high-risk patients and to train dietetic interns.

Other resources that can be used to achieve consistency in the provision of inpatient nutrition care include *Nutrition and Diagnosis-Related Care* and *The Science and Practice of Nutrition Support: A Case-Based Core Curriculum* (15,16). In the near future, ADA plans to publish an MNT protocol for inpatient enteral nutrition support. Until this and other national inpatient MNT protocols are available, dietitians can access existing protocols, or they can use the strategies defined in the ADA publication *Developing and Validating Evidence-Based Guides for Practice: A Tool Kit for Dietetics Professionals* to develop their own evidence-based protocols (17).

Application in the Outpatient Setting

In the outpatient setting, dietitians can use the *American Dietetic Association Medical Nutrition Therapy Evidence-Based Guides for Practice* (9) as the basis for outcomes data collection. The "Progress Note" form that is part of each guide serves dual roles: (1) documentation of client goals, MNT provided, and outcomes, and (2) use in data collection in an outcomes project.

In an outcomes project, the data collected during assessment and monitoring of individual clients must be aggregated and analyzed at the group level. Each MNT Guide includes spreadsheets and templates that can be used to compile and summarize the data for clinic patients with the same diagnosis.

An essential component of both outpatient documentation and outcomes monitoring is tracking the amount of MNT time provided. In an outcomes project, MNT is the intervention being tested. To determine its impact, the amount or dose of MNT provided must be known. Tracking MNT time allows a link to be drawn between the clinical and behavioral changes observed and the MNT intervention. It also allows observation of a dose effect—that is, evaluation of the amount of change in the outcomes when different amounts of MNT are provided.

Evaluation of clinical and behavioral data and data on the amount of MNT intervention provided is also an important aspect of monitoring staffing effectiveness. If desired aggregate outcomes are not being achieved, one factor to evaluate is adequacy of staffing. An evaluation of outcomes data also may determine that staff members do not have the laboratory results and physical measurements they need to assess patients' progress with MNT. In this case, performance improvement activities can be directed toward reducing the variation in monitoring and obtaining the needed laboratory results and physical measurements.

In the outpatient setting, outcomes data can be used to negotiate coverage for MNT by third party payers. Existing payer contracts may be revised to include coverage for MNT, and RDs may be listed as covered providers. These changes require collaboration with personnel in the facility and payer contract offices.

REFERENCES

1. Definition of productivity. WordNet Web site. Available at: *www.cogsci.princeton.edu/cgi-bin/webwn*. Accessed February 26, 2004.

2. Joint Commission on Accreditation of Healthcare Organizations. *Staffing Effectiveness in Hospitals*. Oakbrook Terrace, Ill: Joint Commission Resources; 2003.

3. Smith PC, Kendall LM, Hulin CL. *The Measurement of Satisfaction and Retirement: A Strategy for the Study of Attitudes*. Chicago, Ill: Rand McNally; 1969.

4. Smith PC. *Revised Job Description Index*. Bowling Green, Ohio: Department of Psychology, Bowling Green University; 1985.

5. Dalton S, Gilbride JA, Russo L, Vergis L. Job satisfaction of clinical, community, and long-term-care dietitians in New York City. *J Am Diet Assoc*. 1993; 93:184–188.

6. Agriesti-Johnson C, Broski D. Job satisfaction of dietitians in the United States. *J Am Diet Assoc*. 1982;82:555–559.

7. Mortensen JK, Nyland NK, Fullmer S, Eggett DL. Professional involvement is associated with increased job satisfaction among dietitians. *J Am Diet Assoc*. 2002;102:1452–1454.

8. Bryk JA, Soto TK. Report on the 1999 Membership Database of the American Dietetic Association. *J Am Diet Assoc*. 2001;101:947–953.

9. *American Dietetic Association Medical Nutrition Therapy Evidence-Based Guides for Practice* [CD-ROMs]. Chicago, Ill: American Dietetic Association; 2002.

10. Looking at staffing effectiveness. *Joint Commission Benchmark*. 2003;5(2):1–4.

11. Joint Commission on Accreditation of Healthcare Organizations. *Tools for Performance Measurement in Health Care: A Quick Reference Guide*. Oakbrook Terrace, Ill: Joint Commission Resources; 2002.

12. Gray GE, Gray LK. Evidence-based medicine: applications in dietetic practice. *J Am Diet Assoc*. 2002;102:1263–1271.

13. Haynes RB. Of studies, summaries, synopses, and systems: the "4S" evolution of services for finding current best evidence. *ACP J Club*. 2001;134:A11-A13.

14. Greer N, Mosser G, Logan G, Wagstrom Halaas G. A practical approach to evidence grading. *Jt Comm J Qual Improv*. 2000;26:700–712.

15. Escott-Stump S. *Nutrition and Diagnosis-Related Care*. Baltimore, Md: Williams & Wilkins; 1998.

16. American Society for Parenteral and Enteral Nutrition. *The Science and Practice of Nutrition Support: A Case-Based Core Curriculum.* Dubuque, Iowa: Kendall/Hunt; 2002.

17. Splett PL. *Developing and Validating Evidence-Based Guides for Practice: A Tool Kit for Dietetics Professionals.* Chicago, Ill: American Dietetic Association; 1999.

ADDITIONAL RESOURCES

American Dietetic Association. *Linking Research to Dietetics Practice: An Introduction* [CD-ROM]. Chicago, Ill: American Dietetic Association Publication; 2003.

Ireton-Jones CS, Gottschlich MM, Bell SJ. *Practice-Oriented Nutrition Research: An Outcomes Measurement Approach.* Gaithersburg, Md: Aspen Publishers; 1998.

Monsen ER, ed. *Research: Successful Approaches.* 2nd ed. Chicago, Ill: American Dietetic Association; 2003.

CHAPTER 6

Clinical Nutrition Staffing: Sharing Information

THE ONGOING CHALLENGE

After all the plans have been developed, all the data collected, and all the reports generated, the key to effective clinical nutrition staffing is finding and keeping the right people for the work that needs to be done. As managers know, this activity presents, and probably always will present, an ongoing challenge. It is important work because of the impact of staffing issues (ie, number of staff members, their skill mix and competencies, and turnover) on the quality and cost of health care and on patient safety.

This chapter differs from the previous five chapters. Instead of providing new concepts and forms to use, it focuses on sharing information from available resources, including clinical nutrition managers (CNMs) who are working in today's health care environment and handling staffing issues day in and day out. To obtain insight into staffing issues and the solutions being implemented to address them, CNMs were asked a series of questions about clinical nutrition staffing through a survey that was posted to the Clinical Nutrition Management dietetic practice group electronic mailing list (Spring 2003). Twenty-seven CNMs responded to the initial survey. Ten of these CNMs responded to a second set of questions via e-mail correspondence with the author.

> **Important note:** Responses from this sample of CNMs should be interpreted with caution, because no attempt was made to select a representative sample of CNMs based on facility size, location, acuity, or any other criteria, and the number of CNMs who responded is small. In addition, not all CNMs answered every survey question.

The answers from both the survey and the e-mail correspondences provide a snapshot of options for readers who are facing staffing issues at their own worksites. The CNMs who shared their information and strategies for this chapter obviously are striving to build winning workplaces.

AUTHOR SURVEY ON CLINICAL NUTRITION STAFFING

Twenty-three of the CNMs who responded to the survey work at single-site acute care facilities ranging in size from 80 beds to 800 beds. Four CNMs have multisite management responsibilities at facilities ranging from 50 beds to 200 beds. The CNMs were asked a series of questions about patient care and staffing practices. Table 6.1 shows the responses to each question. As might be expected, registered dietitian (RD) staffing at the facilities where the CNMs work varied considerably, although no attempt was made to correlate facility size with staffing level. The range of distribution of RD positions at the 26 facilities for which data are available was 1.0 to 11.25. The middle of the range, or median number, of full-time equivalents (FTEs) was 5.6. Thirteen CNMs provided data on outpatient RD staffing. Outpatient FTEs ranged from 0.4 to 8.1, with a median of 1.9 FTEs.

Twenty-four CNMs responded with information on dietetic technician staffing. Of these CNMs, 17 had dietetic technicians working in their facilities, whereas 7 did not. At the 17 sites with dietetic technicians, FTEs ranged from 1.0 to 6.6, with a median of 2.0 FTEs.

The CNMs were asked their opinions on anticipated staffing changes that would affect dietitians and dietetic technicians. Their responses, shown in Figure 6.1, indicate that most CNMs expect either no change from present levels of staff or an increase.

Next, the CNMs were asked about their experiences in recruiting and retaining clinical nutrition staff. Specifically, they were asked how much of a problem they have had with recruiting and retention in general (see Figure 6.2 for responses), recruiting experienced clinical nutrition staff (Figure 6.3), retention of entry-level and experienced clinical nutrition staff (Figure 6.4), recruiting specialized clinical nutrition staff (eg, certified nutrition support dietitians, certified diabetes educators, pediatric RDs, and renal RDs) (Figure 6.5), and recruiting diverse clinical nutrition staff (Figure 6.6).

Table 6.1   Patient Care and Staffing Practices

Question	No. of Yes Responses
Have a dietetics internship?	0
Affiliated with a dietetics internship?	21
Dietitian(s) does nutrition screening?	6
Dietetic technician(s) does nutrition screening?	15
Dietetic technician(s) participates in patient care?	13
Have a career ladder for dietitians?	5
Have defined an advanced-practice role for dietitians?	6
Have part-time dietitians on staff?	25
Have initiated job sharing for dietitians?	13

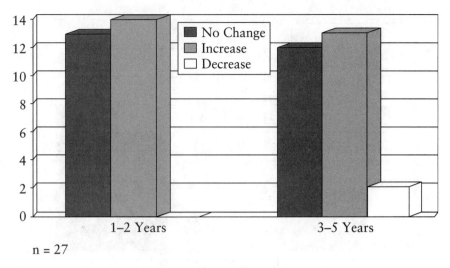

n = 27

Figure 6.1 CNMs' expectations for staffing changes over 5 years.

Recruiting Issues

The CNMs were asked their opinions on the barriers to recruiting clinical nutrition staff. Their responses are presented in Figure 6.7. They appear to perceive salary as the largest barrier, with type of work, inability to pay professional memberships, and inability to pay registration to professional meetings perceived as lesser barriers. Benefits and having paid time off to attend professional meetings are not perceived as barriers. These CNMs may be able to provide paid time off for attending meetings, thus removing this barrier.

Retention Issues

The CNMs also were asked their perceived barriers to staff retention. Their responses are presented in Figure 6.8. The CNMs appear to

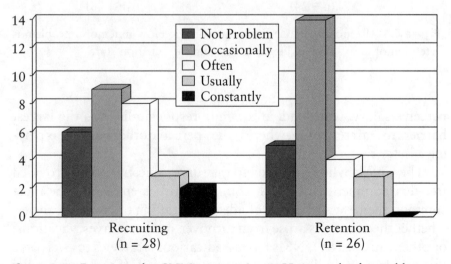

Figure 6.2 Responses by CNMs to question 1: How much of a problem are recruiting and retention of clinical nutrition staff?

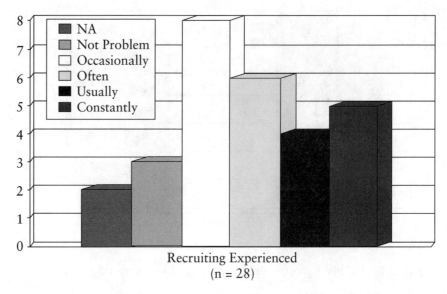

Figure 6.3 Responses by CNMs to question 2: How much of a problem is recruiting experienced clinical nutrition staff? CNMs who do not require RDs to have experience before hiring them into positions were asked to select the "not applicable" (NA) response.

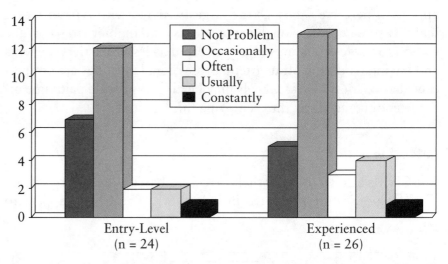

Figure 6.4 Responses by CNMs to question 3: How much of a problem is retention of entry-level and experienced clinical nutrition staff?

perceive salary, workload, and family responsibilities as the largest barriers to staff retention, whereas they perceive other barriers as playing a lesser role.

The CNMs who responded to the survey questions also provided free-text comments, in which common themes emerged. The most common theme was the lack of adequate staffing to cover vacancies, whether the vacancies arose from turnover, medical leaves, vacations, or other causes. The CNMs have used various strategies to overcome this problem, including cross-training existing staff to provide relief coverage, job partnering with cross-training on the units of partner

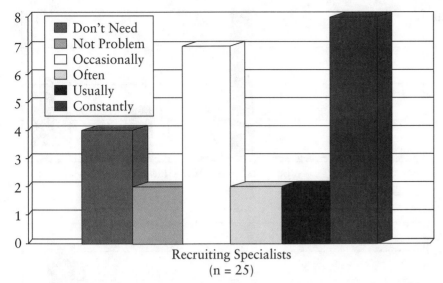

Figure 6.5 Responses by CNMs to question 4: How much of a problem is recruiting specialized clinical nutrition staff?

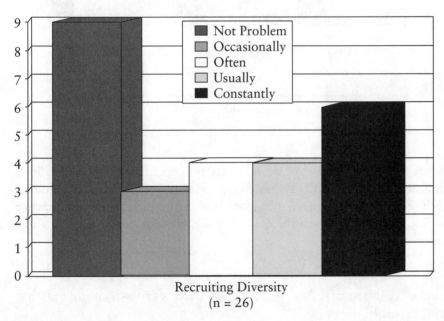

Figure 6.6 Responses by CNMs to question 5: How much of a problem is recruiting diverse clinical nutrition staff?

RDs, using temporary RDs, and having an on-call RD pool from which to pull staff as needed.

A second common theme was an inability to recruit and hire specialized RDs, such as RDs who specialize in nutrition support, neonatal intensive care nutrition, pediatrics, and niches like bone marrow transplant and eating disorders. A strategy commonly used to overcome this problem is to place staff who lack the needed knowledge and skills in these positions—whether by transferring existing staff or hiring new staff—and to provide on-the-job training to obtain the desired

Manager Attitudes and Skills for a Winning Workplace

Clinical nutrition managers set the stage for the teams they manage. Ongoing assessment and building of winning attitudes and skills help ensure that staff find the support they need. Winning workplace attitudes and skills for managers include the following.

Attitudes

- A positive outlook and optimism about the future of clinical nutrition
- Taking action—being proactive in identifying and solving problems
- A willingness to challenge the status quo
- A desire for inclusiveness and involvement of staff in decision making
- Comfort with diversity—encouraging divergent viewpoints
- A belief in empowering staff
- A willingness to let go of control and to delegate authority
- A belief in the importance of balance between work and personal life
- A willingness to share the limelight and let staff take credit for successes achieved

Skills

- Setting direction for a strong, visible clinical nutrition presence in the organization
- Leading teams and being a team member
- Acquiring resources to support staff and programs
- Being creative—able to construct meaningful roles that are appropriate to staff knowledge and skills and to enhance the time staff members spend with patients and their families
- Building relationships
- Seeking partnerships with staff to develop collegiality and respect
- Building connections—establishing links with other departments and fostering opportunities for friendship and socializing within the department
- Listening
- Communicating clear expectations and accountabilities
- Handling underperformers effectively
- Being a role model and mentor

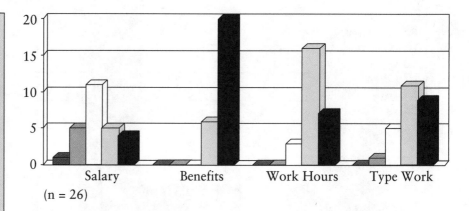

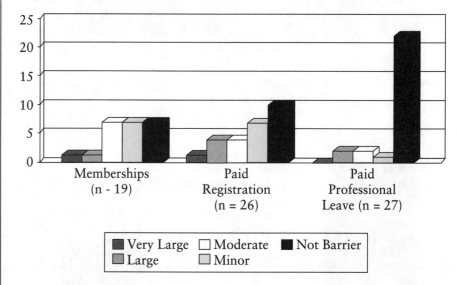

Figure 6.7 CNMs' views of the magnitudes of specific barriers to recruiting clinical nutrition staff. CNMs were given a list of barriers and asked to rate each one in terms of perceived magnitude of the barrier in their own practice setting. The bars represent the number of CNMs who chose each magnitude descriptor.

level of competency. Another strategy used is cross-training existing staff on multiple units.

A third theme that emerged from the comments was heavy staff workloads. Although the CNMs offered some suggestions, such as using technology to streamline work processes, their comments expressed frustration with this problem more often than answers. Related to this frustration was their difficulty in justifying either additional staff or higher salaries.

The final common theme was an inability to recruit dietetic technicians. Although some CNMs are able to be affiliated with local training programs for dietetic technicians or to access training for existing staff members through distance learning programs, most CNMs are not able to find dietetic technicians either in the numbers needed or with the specialized training that could be used in their facilities.

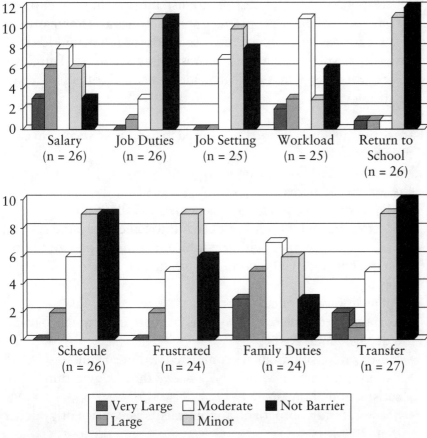

Figure 6.8 CNMs' perceptions of barriers to staff retention. CNMs were given a list of barriers to retaining clinical nutrition staff and asked to rate each one in terms of perceived magnitude of the barrier in their own practice setting. The bars represent the number of CNMs who chose each magnitude descriptor.

AUTHOR SURVEY FOLLOW-UP

In response to the themes that emerged from the CNM electronic mailing list survey, an e-mail questionnaire was sent to the CNMs who indicated that they would be willing to provide additional information. Ten CNMs provided feedback to five additional questions. These questions were specific in their focus and asked for the following:

1. Outcomes the CNMs use to determine success in clinical nutrition staffing.
2. Interventions that managers need to implement to achieve these measures of success.
3. Strategies the CNMs have used to increase clinical nutrition staffing and salaries.
4. Strategies the CNMs have used to increase productivity and achieve workload efficiencies.
5. Strategies the CNMs have used to increase staff retention and job satisfaction.

The responses to each question are listed below in their entirety. Some responses will be appropriate in some settings and not in others. However, because readers have diverse needs and may find ideas in even the simplest of suggestions, all responses are listed. Duplicate responses, when listed, may indicate wider use and usefulness of a particular strategy.

What are the outcomes or end points used to determine success in clinical nutrition staffing?

- Screening 100% of the patients.
- Assessing all patients at risk.
- Meeting time frames for assessments and follow-ups.
- Meeting our continuous quality improvement parameters (eg, patients are assessed within established time frames and notes on patients receiving nothing by mouth are written on day 3 to day 5).
- All positions are filled.
- Turnover rate is below 14%—this is an organizational goal and a departmental goal.
- Nutrition consultations are completed within 24 hours—"24/7."
- Patient satisfaction with services—we do our own outpatient satisfaction phone surveys.
- Show rate for outpatient appointments is consistently higher than 70%.
- Enteral and parenteral data collection for medical staff show that best practices are consistently used.
- Receipt of unsolicited feedback from other departments on the job my staff members are doing and the outcomes that are achieved.

Hospital:

- Ninety-five percent of nutrition assessments are completed on time.
- Seventy percent patient care time, 30% non—patient care time for RDs, and the reverse for technicians.
- Staffing ratio of approximately 70 patients per nonacute RD and approximately 40 patients per RD working in acute care areas.
- Reduction in length of stay via use of indirect calorimetry measures early in the treatment of eating disorders, wounds, and so on.

Clinic:

- A third of the available appointments are open within 21 working days.
- Improvement in HgbA1C levels.
- Chart audits are at or above our threshold—we track numbers of assessments and education consultations, as well as percentage increase in volumes.

- Hours per unit of service within our target.
- Units of service, measured as meals, at target.
- All high-risk patients are assessed no later than hospital day 2 or 24 hours after being identified at nutritional risk. I verify this by reviewing charts and information in our automated diet office system.
- Identification of goals and outcomes in chart documentation and determination of whether they are met.
- Compliance with our standards of care, which include documentation and education, monitored through audits.
- Use of diagnostic (disease-specific) care plans.
- Appropriate use of dietitians' time in clinical and nonclinical activities, determined from daily productivity reports and monthly summaries. (Our documented time every month runs very close to 100%.)
- Percentage of patients seen within our policy and procedure guidelines.
- Positive outcomes for nutrition support patients (eg, improvement in lab results, discontinuation of ventilatory support, discontinuation of nutrition support, or transition from parenteral to enteral nutrition support).
- Meeting our standards-of-care time lines (eg, follow up on high-risk patients every 3 days and follow up on consultations within 24 hours).
- Limited use of overtime.

What do managers need to do to achieve these outcomes or "measures of success"?
- Monitor indicators throughout the year.
- Measure productivity for direct patient care.
- Identify trends in the data to identify problems.
- Inform staff when there are discrepancies.
- Prepare quality improvement reports.
- Work overtime. (Because they are all salaried, I ask the dietitians to report the amount of time worked beyond scheduled hours to complete their duties, as well as any clinical care activities that are deferred until the next day due to lack of time. Data can be used to justify additional staff if existing staff are unable to complete their workload in approved time frames. Or data may indicate a need to rework the system to improve efficiency.)
- Share data with staff.
- Set clear expectations.
- Provide a solid orientation for new employees and employees who are transferred into new jobs.
- Define policies and procedures in writing.
- Obtain staff feedback on process improvement.
- Reward staff and provide recognition for a job well done (not necessarily monetary rewards).

- Interact with staff in other departments and with physicians to obtain their perceptions and feedback.
- Establish standards of care that are clear.
- Make the standards of care available.
- Standardize documentation and use electronic charting, if available.
- Measure performance consistently.
- Keep records of productivity.
- Measure increases or decreases in productivity.
- Balance staff workloads.
- Train staff.
- Closely monitor compliance with budgeted hours and actual worked hours.
- Monitor the census.
- Complete chart reviews and periodic studies.
- Require RDs to document specific cases where cost savings have occurred or length of stay has been decreased due to their intervention or recommendations.
- Monitor the parts of the nutrition care process completed by other members of the health care team.
- Educate the nursing and physician staffs, as well as the RD staff.
- Get support from staff members.
- Involve staff in audits and reviews.
- Solicit staff input for solutions to problems.

What specific strategies have you used to increase your clinical nutrition staffing and salaries?
- We had to use our direct patient care data to demonstrate staff productivity.
- When we did not meet our quality improvement goals for timeliness of assessments and follow-ups, we were able to justify additional staffing.
- To date I have not been able to increase staffing level or salaries. I have worked to maintain state licensure fees at their current amount.

I do the following:
- Use volume statistics.
- Demonstrate requirements when planning programs.
- Monitor the budget closely.
- Calculate costs of hiring staff with the skill mix needed.
- Work with human resources (HR) staff members to evaluate the annual salary survey data they receive for our region of the country.
- Collaborate with our recruiter to achieve appropriate starting pay for new hires (ie, I obtain the best salary quotes possible before staff members are hired).
- Keep administrators aware of nutrition standards.

- Provide performance measurement data to administrators on an ongoing basis.
- Demonstrate how staffing levels are essential to compliance with Medicare, state health department, and Joint Commission on Accreditation of Healthcare Organizations (JCAHO) regulations, standards, and requirements.
- Provide evidence of staff efficiency and effectiveness in meeting the standards, along with revenue and expense data and outcome reports.
- Collect and report data based on productivity reports.
- I have not been able to increase salaries, since our salaries are comparable to those at other area facilities.
- Since our census has gone down, we are working to maintain our staffing. We recently gave up a 0.7-FTE technician.
- We are at "market" for salaries in our area.
- Conduct studies on patients at high nutritional risk.
- Conduct time management studies using relative value units to determine the time required to complete specific direct care tasks and the number of tasks that need to be done.
- Notify the HR department when there are problems recruiting staff.
- Provide special premium pay as needed when retention is a problem.
- We have not technically increased clinical staffing. I do have one 32-hour-per-week outpatient RD who agreed to work on a new menu for the management team during the 8 hours she had available each week. She has since become invaluable to the team, and they want this additional 8 hours to become permanent.
- We have not had any increases in salaries beyond our annual raises.
- Our staffing is primarily based on comparisons of census among the hospitals in our region that are owned by our hospital corporation. Each time I have needed to increase hours or positions, I have had to do a comparison of services provided and RD-to-patient ratios within our region. I usually include a few hospitals that are not part of the corporation, although our HR department relies solely on internal comparisons.
- I have not been successful in getting salaries increased.
- Make sure staff members have multiple skills, so when areas for growth and increased revenue are identified (eg, expansion of the outpatient nutrition clinic), there is support for hiring additional staff.
- Conduct patient satisfaction surveys to support growth of new services.
- Our salary schedule is based on years of experience. We've benchmarked our salaries with those of other area facilities and met with our HR department to discuss the costs associated with retaining experienced staff. In spite of the benchmarking, our

salaries for entry-level staff are not always enough to retain them. HR agreed that to retain these individuals, we needed to move them beyond the salary step that corresponds with their years of experience.

What specific strategies have you used to increase productivity (ie, to achieve workload efficiencies)?

- We use evaluation of direct patient care percentages as a criteria in our annual performance evaluations for RDs. We require that 70% of the inpatient RDs' time be spent in direct care and 50% of outpatient RDs' time be spent in direct care.
- If someone is not functioning at an appropriate level, we will adjust the workload among staff.
- Setting targets for increased productivity.
- Recognition of staff members who have achieved higher productivity.
- Discussion of quality and service data and benchmark comparisons with staff, building their support for goals.
- Automation whenever possible to cut down on paper handling.
- Cross-training.
- Use of RD-DTR teams.
- Continual reevaluation of the work environment and client population data to identify changes that indicate a need for staff modifications.
- Peer audits of documentation.
- Development of standards of care that are clear and available.
- Standardized charting.
- Consistent performance measurement.
- Electronic charting. (This is a "biggie.")
- Staffing is flexed based on the census.
- Inpatient RDs counsel additional outpatients when time permits.
- Clinical staff do not have any operations responsibilities. They are expected to spend 80% to 85% of their time in patient care. This is explained to all applicants during the interview process.
- We share data among staff, and as a result, everyone knows how many high-risk patients each RD has and also the average amount of time each works daily.
- Most staff are cross-trained to work in a variety of situations. Several staff members can teach each class we offer, and they are all familiar with each other's floors.
- We are an acute care facility and see only moderate- to high-risk patients.
- I monitor the acuity of the patients receiving nutrition care and regularly refine our screening process based on these reviews. For instance, I recently increased the age we use for defining "geriatric" for our surgery patients. I evaluated the patients the RDs had assessed who were over age 65. In doing this, I found that most of these patients did not have other nutrition risk cri-

teria and therefore were at low risk. At that point, we increased our age for "geriatric" to 80. I continued monitoring the nutrition risk level of patients being referred for nutrition assessment and determined that many patients did not need a full assessment. As a result, we changed our referral process from requiring one nutrition risk criterion for nutrition assessment to requiring two criteria.

- Time studies to define average time for specific tasks.
- Benchmarking to compare measurements with those used at other facilities.
- Standardization of clinical notes.
- Charting by exception.
- Identification of the acuity levels of each patient unit and assignment of staffing based on this acuity level and the unit's average patient census.

What strategies have you used to increase staff retention and job satisfaction?

- Although my staff is salaried, I do not want them to work significantly more than 40 hours on a regular basis.
- Job sharing.
- Increasing the maximum salary for RDs from 50% above the minimum to 75% above the minimum.
- I use motivators that do not cost any money, due to the cost containment philosophy of my facility. For example, I wrote each of my own employees a personal note thanking them for their extra hard work during a summer when we were short staffed. I presented the notes at what I called a "mandatory meeting" (party).
- I give personal recognition for doing a good job.
- As a manager, I am accessible to staff when they need me via phone, pager, and e-mail.
- I practice participative management as part of our service excellence initiative.
- I meet with new staff members 30 days and 60 days from their hire dates, taking time to sit and chat about how they are progressing. We do this over a private lunch.
- I continually work at the management level to recognize staff and promote their professional image to others in our facility.
- I am proactive in addressing sources of dissatisfaction identified by staff members.
- I always make time for staff, no matter how busy I am.
- We have a partnership council structure that ensures that all staff members have a voice in decisions.
- We have developed a work team that focuses on planning activities designed to recognize staff achievements and to facilitate more socialization. Since we have several regional sites, this is important.

- We use special note cards to let others know that they are appreciated and do good work.
- We have monthly continuing education opportunities and have appointed a person to coordinate continuing education hours.
- We practice the *FISH!* philosophy [named for the philosophy of teamwork and customer service that was developed at the Pike Place Fish Market in Seattle].
- Just for fun, we pass a birthday mug filled with goodies. We also use the mug for other special occasions and accomplishments.
- We set aside time for special recognitions during our monthly staff meetings. Recognition is an item on our meeting agenda.
- To enhance communication, we use a shared on-line directory on which we post all patient education materials, care standards, meeting agendas and minutes, calendars of events, and staff schedules.
- We use of staff satisfaction surveys to identify staff needs and then work to meet these needs.
- On a quarterly basis, and more often when possible, I meet face to face with each RD in what I call "touching base" meetings. RDs can say whatever they want to, and I don't bring up anything negative. During these meetings, I ask for feedback on my performance as a manager and for suggestions on ways that I can do a better job. This has really helped with nonprofessional staff.
- I encourage staff to be accountable for their work, and I involve them in the hospital service lines. This helps bring their value within the institution to the forefront. Our retention is good.
- Flex time.
- Approval of requests for time off, when possible.
- Appropriate management style: I avoid micromanaging, treat staff like the professionals they are, and give them accountability and responsibility.
- During orientation, each new staff member receives a notebook containing very detailed information. This information helps them acclimate to their area of responsibility.
- I have been in my position as CNM for 2 years now and have had very little turnover. I think part of the reason for this low turnover is that I work to maintain an open, honest relationship with the dietitians. I make them feel like I am a part of their team and not necessarily their "boss." I cover one patient floor, because the hospital has had higher than 100% occupancy for most of this year. I demonstrate that I am always willing to roll up my sleeves and help get the job done.
- I have hired a team of RDs who work very well together. During interviews, I look for specific interpersonal competencies that are important for success at my facility.
- I have worked to build a strong relationship between the RDs and the management team. Before I came to this facility, there

was a lot of "us" versus "them" between these two groups, which resulted in a difficult working relationship. The relationship has improved, and now the dietitians feel more like they are part of the department team. They feel that they have some say in what happens in our food service.

- Participation in decision making.
- Staff-driven projects.
- Creative National Nutrition Month activities.
- Flexibility with schedules and flex scheduling. I do my best to say yes to schedule requests!
- I try to accommodate assignment preferences.
- I really trust my staff with their schedules. I have asked that they keep me informed when they have off-site appointments, are away from the facility for a few hours, and work earlier or later than scheduled. I had one staff member who left for a few hours during the day to take a scuba class at the local Y and made up her time by working early and late on the day of her class. My stipulation is that the RDs work with their peers to make sure unit coverage isn't negatively affected.

Revisions in the Accreditation Process

APPENDIX A.   REVISIONS IN THE ACCREDITATION PROCESS

In 1999 the Joint Commission on Accreditation of Healthcare Organizations (JCAHO) issued a white paper entitled *The Possible Accreditation Process Circa 2003,* in which it outlined a vision for a possible future accreditation process. (1) In the paper, JCAHO described its intent to create a valid and relevant accreditation process for health care facilities that relies on a model that is "more data-driven, less predictable and more customized to the individual organization" (1). Since that time, JCAHO has engaged in activities to bring the vision to reality and consequently launched the new model in 2004 (2).

A component of the new model is the midcycle facility self-assessment. Each facility is expected to complete a periodic performance review of its compliance with all applicable standards by the 18-month point in its triennial accreditation cycle and to provide JCAHO with an attestation to this compliance. When the self-assessment reveals noncompliance or a lower score than the full score allowed, the facility must choose one of several options: (1) to submit a plan of action, a report outlining actions taken to achieve compliance and measures of success (MOS) that validate resolution of identified problems; (2) to complete the plan of action, attest to its completion, but refrain from submitting it to JCAHO and provide the MOS to surveyors during the triennial survey; or (3) to undergo a shortened on-site survey at the midpoint of its accreditation cycle, develop a plan of action to address any problems identified, and provide the MOS to surveyors at the full survey. JCAHO staff members are available to review the plans of action with facility staff after submission (if they are submitted, as in the first option) or via telephone or electronic communication (if they are not submitted, as in the second option).

The triennial survey itself has been revised to include four components. The first component is the setting aside of time slots for discussion and consultation. Topics for discussion include patient safety; the use of performance improvement data such as that used for core performance measurements and the analysis of staffing, emergency preparedness, and other topics that JCAHO determines to be relevant at the time of the survey. The second component of the survey is a validation exercise on the standards for which compliance plans were submitted and a review of compliance with a randomly selected sample of other standards.

JCAHO has called the process it uses to determine the focus of the on-site triennial survey its *priority focus process.* Using a Web-based automated program, JCAHO integrates and analyzes data from a variety of sources using established rules and algorithms. The result of data integration and analysis is identification of a list of facility-specific priority clinical processes to be reviewed during the survey and generation of a demographic description of services and populations served. The description is used to select charts for review during the triennial survey.

The method JCAHO uses for determining compliance with selected standards during a survey is known as *tracer methodology*. *Patient tracers* are several patients selected by the surveyors at the beginning of the survey for tracing through the facility's care processes. Data gathered prior to the survey, including data from the on-line application submitted by the facility, are used as the basis for the random selection. Visits to patient care units, departments, and other sites—the third component of the survey—follow the same flow sequence as that actually experienced by the patients who are selected. Staff in these areas are interviewed about the care provided to patients and relevant standards. The fourth component of the triennial survey includes the leadership interview, along with opening and closing conferences.

JCAHO also uses *systems tracers* to analyze key operational systems that directly affect the quality and safety of patient care. Time is set aside during the survey for in-depth discussions on these priority topics.

Another change that was implemented in 2002 as part of the new vision for the accreditation process was the revision of surveyor procedures. All surveyors are now required to pass a general certification examination, and as of 2003, each surveyor is required to pass a program-specific certification examination. Recertification is required at 5-year intervals. Surveyors have been given intense training on systems theory, organizational behavior, and evaluation techniques. Beginning in 2002, JCAHO implemented a program of surveyor observation by supervisors and mentors in order to provide on-site surveyor evaluation and to identify additional training needs.

The final piece of the program for surveyors is the creation of a database of surveyor profiles that includes scores and recommendations given for each standard by the surveyor, aggregate feedback from the postsurvey evaluations of facilities surveyed by the surveyor, and aggregate data on successful revision requests as a percentage of total survey reports completed by the surveyor. A facility submits revision requests to appeal an adverse score given by a surveyor during a survey; successful revision requests were successfully appealed. Surveyor profiles are used for quality control and identification of training needs.

The impact of these changes will be felt over time. However, JCAHO has made it very clear that it expects to use data-driven processes and technology in the accreditation process. It also intends for the process to involve continual submission of data rather than "ramping up" (ie, relatively low-key operations for the first half of the triennial cycle followed by frenzied preparation for an upcoming survey 12 to 18 months in advance of it). To accomplish all this, JCAHO surveys after 2006 will be unannounced. They will take place during a 2- to 4-year window following the facility's prior triennial survey.

During 2004 and 2005, announced triennial surveys and randomly selected unannounced surveys continue. However, JCAHO has revised the performance areas evaluated during the unannounced surveys. Four critical focus areas—staffing, infection control, medication management, and facility-specific initiatives to meet the national patient safety goals—are fixed performance areas that will be assessed. Variable performance areas that are part of these surveys will be based on prioritized, facility-specific critical focus areas.

Nutrition managers and staff need to be aware of the changes that have been outlined and of all future changes as they unfold. They also need to use technology to gather and analyze performance and staffing data, in line with the directions set by JCAHO.

REFERENCES

1. Joint Commission on Accreditation of Healthcare Organizations. The Possible Accreditation Process Circa 2003 [1999 white paper], as quoted in The Accreditation Process Circa 2004 (p.1). Available at: *http://www.jcaho.org*. Accessed January 15, 2003.
2. Joint Commission on Accreditation of Healthcare Organizations. The Accreditation Process Circa 2004. Available at: *http://www.jcaho.org*. Accessed January 15, 2003.

Assessing Staffing Needs: Worksheets

APPENDIX B.1 FACILITY OVERVIEW

Facility _____

Completed by _____   Date_____

Item	Information	Source
Type of facility		
Community setting		
Geographic area served		
Number and type of beds	Adult patients: Intensive care_____ Medicine _____ Surgical _____ Pediatric patients: Neonatal intensive care _____ Pediatric intensive care _____ Medicine _____ Surgical _____ Obstetrics: _____ Extended care: Rehab _____ Subacute _____	
Number of units and buildings	Units _____ Buildings _____	
Acuity level		
Average length of stay		
Relation to other hospitals		
Financial management		

Item	Information	Source
Physician relationship(s) to facility		
Facility mission		
Vision		
Annual goals and facility initiatives		
Budget priorities		
Long-range plans and goals		
Community alliances		
Patient populations • Ages • Diagnoses and conditions		

(continues)

144ACHIEVING EXCELLENCE

APPENDIX B.1   (*continued*)

Item	Information	Source
• Services, programs, and procedures		

Item	Description
Facility characteristics that affect staffing	

Instructions:

This form should be completed by a manager or other assigned staff using the directions provided in Facility Overview section of Chapter 1.

APPENDIX B.2   DEPARTMENT OVERVIEW*

Department _____

Completed by _____   Date_____

*Attach copies of current organizational charts for facility and department.

Item	Information	Source
Relation of clinical nutrition service to foodservice	Part of same department _____ Separate departments _____	

Department management structure	Self-operated _____ Contract managed_____
	
	Clinical nutrition director or manager:
	
	   Yes____ No ___
	
	Manager/director responsibilities:
	
	   Single department _____
	
	   Multiple nutrition departments _____
	
	   Multiple departments plus nutrition
	
	   department _____	

Clinical nutrition staffing	Clinical nutrition staff: (Check if yes) Hospital employees _____ Contract management employees _____ Unionized _____ RDs exempt _____ Career ladder _____	

Dietetic technicians	Working in facility:
	
	   Yes _____ No _____
	Involved in clinical nutrition care:
	
	   Yes_____ No_____
	DTRs _____ Non-DTRs _____	

Applications of technology in patient care • Facility-wide		
• In the department		

APPENDIX B.2   (*continued*)

Item	Information	Source
Role with dietetics interns and students		
Annual goals • Department • Clinical nutrition unit		
Long-range plans and goals		
Menu system		
Food production and delivery		
Settings for nutrition care delivery	Check, as appropriate: Inpatient _____ Outpatient clinics _____ Home health care_____ Subacute care _____ Long-term care _____ Other _____ (describe)	
Patient care teams and RD roles		

Item	Description
Department characteristics that affect staffing	

Instructions:

This form should be completed by a manager or other assigned staff using the directions provided in Facility Overview section of Chapter 1.

APPENDIX B.3   BALANCED SCORECARD APPROACH TO STRATEGIC PLANNING

Mission:

_____

_____

_____

_____

Vision:

_____

_____

_____

_____

Priorities for performance areas:

    1. Internal processes

    2. Finances

    3. Customers

    4. Innovation and learning

Gap Analysis

	Performance Areas			
	Internal Processes	Finances	Customers	Innovation and Learning
Current status				
Desired status				
Strategies for moving from current to desired status				
Key performance indicators				

Instructions:

This form should be completed by the manager and other assigned staff on an annual basis. Refer to explanation provided in "Department Overview" section of Chapter 1.

Developing a Staffing Plan: Worksheets

APPENDIX C.1   ADMISSION NUTRITIONAL RISK AUDIT

Unit _____   Auditor _____

Date	Total Number of Admissions	Low or No Risk	Moderate Risk	High Risk
Totals				
%				

Instructions:

1. Complete an audit for a 7-day period. Staff on each unit should complete audits for the same 1-week interval. When possible, complete audits for 1-week intervals in each 3-month quarter of the year.
2. List the following data in the correct column, by date:
   • Total number of patients admitted to the unit.
   • Number of patients at each level of nutritional risk. Adjust the names and numbers of risk categories to correspond with facility procedures.
3. Add each column to obtain the total number of patients admitted to the unit for a 1-week period and the total numbers of patients in each nutritional risk category.
4. Calculate the percentage of patients in each risk category:
   (Total number of patients in risk category ÷ Total number of patients admitted to unit during 1-week interval) × 100.

Note: See Appendix D.1 for a completed example of this form.

APPENDIX C.2   ADMISSION NUTRITIONAL RISK SUMMARY

Dates of Audit _____ to _____

Unit	Total Number of Admissions	Low or No Risk	Moderate Risk	High Risk
Totals				
%		X	Y	Z

Instructions:

1. List the total numbers of admissions and patients in each category of nutritional risk for each unit.
2. Add each column to obtain the total number of patients admitted to all units for the 1-week period and the total numbers of patients in each nutritional risk category.
3. Calculate the percentage of patients in each risk category for the entire facility:
   (Total number of patients in risk category ÷ Total number of patients admitted to facility during 1-week interval) × 100.
   X = percentage of low-risk patients; Y = percentage of moderate-risk patients; and Z = percentage of high-risk patients.
4. Transfer calculated percentages for X, Y, and Z to two locations in Appendix C.11: Patient Care Staffing Estimates.

Note: See Appendix D.2 for a completed example of this form.

APPENDIX C.3   NUTRITIONAL STATUS—FACILITY PROFILE

Date of Audit _____

Unit	Total Number of Patients	Low or No Risk	Moderate Risk	High Risk
Totals				
%				

Instructions:

1. List the total numbers of patients on each unit in the facility and the numbers of patients in each category of nutritional risk by unit. Add additional lines in the table as needed for additional units.
2. Add each column to obtain the total number of patients on all units on the day of the audit and the total numbers of patients in each nutritional risk category.
3. Calculate the percentage of patients in each risk category for the entire facility:
   (Total number of patients in risk category ÷ Total number of patients hospitalized in facility on the day of the audit) × 100.

APPENDIX C.4 GENERAL NUTRITION CARE TIME AUDIT

Unit _____ Auditor _____ Audit Dates_____ to_____

Patient MR No.	Nutrition Screening			Patient MR No.	Rescreening			Patient MR No.	Nutritional Risk Status Evaluation		
	Start	Stop	Minutes		Start	Stop	Minutes		Start	Stop	Minutes
Total no.		Total time		Total no.		Total time		Total no.		Total time	
		Average				Average				Average	

(*continues*)

APPENDIX C.4   (*continued*)

Unit _____ Auditor _____ Audit Dates_____ to_____

Patient MR No.	NPO and Clear Liquid Monitoring			Patient MR No.	_____			Patient MR No.	_____		
	Start	Stop	Minutes		Start	Stop	Minutes		Start	Stop	Minutes
Total no.		Total time		Total no.		Total time		Total no.		Total time	
		Average				Average				Average	

Instructions:

1. Choose a week (7 days) when all staff are working (ie, no vacations or other leave are scheduled). Each staff member should complete his/her own audit form.
2. Include data for weekend coverage (ie, staff working the weekend should record data for these days, as well as other days worked during the week). Columns have been included for other unit-based activities that are not listed on the form but are completed by clinical nutrition staff at the facility.

3. Record the medical record number (MR No.) for each patient for whom nutrition care is provided during the audit period.

4. List the start and stop times for each of the listed activities completed for each patient. For example: Nutrition screening started at 10:00 a.m. and stopped at 10:12 a.m.

5. Calculate and list the minutes spent on each activity for each patient.

6. Record the total number of patients for whom each activity was completed during the audit period in the shaded "Total no." boxes on the next-to-last line of the form.

7. Add the total number of minutes spent in each activity during the audit period and list this in the shaded "Total time" boxes on the next-to-last line of the form.

8. Calculate the average time spent on each activity by dividing the total number of minutes spent on the activity by the number of patients for that activity. Record the average times for each activity in the shaded boxes on the last line of the form. Transfer data for all audited units to Appendix C.5: General Nutrition Care Time Audit Summary.

Note: See Appendix D.3 for a completed example of this form.

APPENDIX C.5 GENERAL NUTRITION CARE TIME AUDIT SUMMARY

Audit Dates _____ to _____ (7-day interval)

Unit	Nutrition Screening		Rescreening		Nutritional Risk Status Evaluation		NPO and Clear Liquid Monitoring		(Add Other Activities As Needed)	
	Minutes	Patients	Minutes	Patients	Minutes	Patients	Minutes	Patients	Minutes	Patients
Total	Minutes	Patients	Minutes (M-1)	Patients (P-1)	Minutes (M-2)	Patients (P-2)	Minutes (M-3)	Patients (P-3)	Minutes	Patients
Per-patient averages		S		T		U		V		
Annual time estimates		$S \times$ No. of admits		$M\text{-}1 \times 52$		$M\text{-}2 \times 52$		$M\text{-}3 \times 52$		

Instructions:

1. List the units included in the audit in the shaded column on the left of the form.
2. List the total number of minutes spent in each activity for each unit audited from Appendix C.4: General Nutrition Care Time Audit. List the total number of patients for each activity by unit from Appendix C.4. Include data from all staff who worked on each unit during the audit period, including weekends.
3. Add the unit totals to get the facility total of number of minutes for each activity for the audit period (1 week) and the total number of patients for each activity for the audit period.
4. The results for rescreening, nutrition risk status evaluation, and NPO/clear liquid monitoring are assigned codes:
   - M-1 for rescreening time
   - M-2 for nutrition risk status evaluation time
   - M-3 for NPO/clear liquid monitoring time
   - P-1 for rescreening patients
   - P-2 for nutrition risk status evaluation patients
   - P-3 for NPO/clear liquid monitoring patients).
5. Calculate facility's per-patient averages for each activity by dividing total time spent per activity during the audit period by the total number of patients for each activity. A letter code has been assigned to each average:
   - S = average time per nutrition screen
   - T = average time rescreening
   - U = average time per nutrition risk status evaluation
   - V = average time per NPO/clear liquid monitoring.
6. Estimate facility's total annual time for each activity as follows:
   - Nutrition screening = S multiplied by the number of patients admitted to the facility per year. (The number of admissions is obtained from facility reports.) Logic: each patient admitted to the facility must have a nutrition screening.
   - Rescreening = M-1 mulitiplied by 52. Logic: not all patients will need to be rescreened. Assuming that the weekly average time calculated from the audit is representative of a typical week, this number is multiplied by 52 to derive an annual estimate.
   - Nutrition risk evaluation = M-2 multiplied by 52. Assuming that the weekly average time calculated from the audit is representative of a typical week, this number is multiplied by 52 to derive an annual estimate.
   - NPO/clear liquid monitoring = M-3 multiplied by 52. Assuming that the weekly average time calculated from the audit is representative of a typical week, this number is multiplied by 52 to derive an annual estimate.
7. Transfer the annual time estimates for each unit-based activity to the Patient Care Staffing Estimates form in Appendix C.11.

Note: See Appendix D.4 for a completed example of this form.

APPENDIX C.6   ACTIVITY TIME AUDIT—INDIRECT AND NONPATIENT CARE

Unit _____ Auditor _____ Audit Dates _____ to_____

Date	Daily Organizational Activities			Team Rounds			Group Patient Education		
	Start	Stop	Minutes	Start	Stop	Minutes	Start	Stop	Minutes
		Total time			Total time			Total time	

Unit _____ Auditor _____ Audit Dates _____ to_____

Date	Indirect Care Activities			Student Training			Nonpatient Care		
	Start	Stop	Minutes	Start	Stop	Minutes	Start	Stop	Minutes
		Total time			Total time			Total time	

Instructions (for Appendix C.6, pp. 160–161):

1. This form is used to determine the amount of time spent on indirect care and non–patient care activities for a 7-day interval. Each member of the staff should track his/her own information using a separate form.
2. For each day of the audit, record start and stop times for each type of activity listed. Use the information below to determine how to categorize activity types. List activities as many times as they take place (ie, types of activities may be listed more than once per day).
3. Calculate the number of minutes spent on each activity and list this in the column headed "Minutes."
4. Calculate the total minutes for each type of activity by adding the minutes for each activity. List in the unshaded box in the last row on the form.
5. Transfer the data for each staff member participating in the audit to Appendix C.7: Activity Time Audit Summary–Indirect and Nonpatient Care.

Indirect Care Activities:

- Project planning and work time
- Meetings
- Providing and receiving job-related training, including time spent planning training and creating handouts
- Community programs, classes, and support groups
- Performance improvement projects and activities
- Outcomes data collection and related activities
- Research
- Food service activities

Non–Patient Care Time

- Travel time from one work area to another
- Personal breaks
- Delays

Daily Organizational Activities:

- Checking patient lists and generating computer reports
- Planning workload
- Discussions about workload and assignments with other clinical nutrition staff, including providing updates related to days off, weekend coverage, and/or patient transfers
- Updating computer or patient files related to workload
- Email and correspondence
- Telephone calls unrelated to patient care. (calls that are not case management activities)

Team Rounds:

- Bedside rounds and other health care team rounds
- Care planning meetings and conferences
- Discharge planning meetings

Student Training:

- Time spent preparing for, training, providing oversight to, and evaluating dietetic interns and/or students
- Classes taught to dietetic interns, including planning and preparation time
- Classes and programs for other students, including planning and preparation time

Group Patient Care Education:

- Preparation for, conducting, and documenting group nutrition education programs for patients and/or family members

Note: See Appendix D.5 for a completed example of this form.

APPENDIX C.7   ACTIVITY TIME AUDIT SUMMARY—INDIRECT AND NONPATIENT CARE

Audit Dates _____ to _____

(7-day interval)

Staff Name	Daily Organizational Activities	Team Rounds	Group Patient Education	Indirect Care Activities	Student Training	Nonpatient Care
Subtotal	Minutes	Minutes	Minutes	Minutes	Minutes	Minutes
Divide minutes by 60	Hours	Hours	Hours	Hours	Hours	Hours
Adjusted time requirements	Hours	Hours	Hours	Hours	Hours	Hours
Total time/week:	Total time/year:					
Total time/week: Hours	Multiply total time/week by 52.	Hours FTEs				
Add hours for each type of activity.						

Instructions (for Appendix C.7, p. 163):

1. In the left column, list the names of all staff who participated in the audit.
2. Record the number of minutes spent by each staff member on each type of activity, from Appendix C.6: Activity Time Audit-Indirect and Nonpatient Care.
3. Add the minutes in each column to obtain a total number of minutes spent by all staff for each activity. Record the total minutes for each type of activity in the Subtotal row of the form.
4. Convert minutes to hours (divide number of minutes by 60).
5. Make adjustments in time requirements as needed. Refer to Notes below. If no adjustments are needed, the numbers in this row are the same as those on the prior row.
6. Calculate the total hours required per week by adding the number of hours in each box in the Adjusted Time Requirements row. List this total in the second box from the left in the last row on the form.
7. Multiply this number (ie, the total derived in step 6) by 52 to calculate the yearly total for indirect care and non–patient care activities. List in the farthest right unshaded box on the last row of the form.
8. Divide the yearly total in hours by 2,080 to derive the number of FTEs required. List in the same box.

Notes:

- When determining weekly time totals for each activity, evaluate factors that might increase or decrease weekly requirement and make adjustments in totals as appropriate. For example, if dietetics interns are present for three fourths of the year, the required weekly time would need to be adjusted to reflect this. Because of staff involvement in other types of student training, it may not be accurate to adjust the time per week to three fourths of the calculated amount. However, a reduction below the calculated amount will be indicated.
- In lieu of doing an audit, staff can estimate the time spent in each activity. These data can be recorded on the Activity Time Audit Summary, and a final time requirement can be estimated as described above (ie, total time for each activity is determined by adding estimates for each activity for all staff and making any adjustments to reflect variation based on schedules, etc).

Note: See Appendix D.6 for a completed example of this form.

APPENDIX C.8   DIRECT NUTRITION CARE AUDIT—INDIVIDUAL PATIENT

Unit _____   Patient MR No. _____   Nutritional Risk Level _____

Auditor _____   Audit Dates _____ to _____

Date	Nutrition Assessment			Monitoring and Reassessment			Nutrition Education			Nutrition-Drug Interaction Counseling			Case Management—Related Duties			Other		
	Start	Stop	Min	Start	Stop	Min	Start	Stop	Min	Start	Stop	Min	Start	Stop	Min	Start	Stop	Min
Total activity time (min)			(1)			(2)			(3)			(4)			(5)			(6)

Total intervention (min) (Add 1–6)   (7)

Instructions (for Appendix C.8, p. 165):

1. This form is used to determine the amount of time spent in direct care.
2. One form needs to be completed for each patient receiving direct nutrition care during the audit period. For each patient, list at the top of the form the unit, patient's medical record number, and nutrition risk level.
3. Record activities by date. List the start and stop times for each activity performed. Calculate the number of minutes spent in each activity and record for each activity in the shaded columns headed "Min."
4. Add the minutes for each activity and record in the second-to-last row on the form.
   - Box 1 = Total time for nutrition assessment
   - Box 2 = Total time for monitoring and reassessment
   - Box 3 = Total time for nutrition education
   - Box 4 = Total time for nutrient-drug interaction counseling
   - Box 5 = Total time for case management-related duties
   - Box 6 = Total time for other direct care activities (facility-specific)
5. Determine total direct care time for each patient by adding the totals for all activities. List this total in Box 7. Transfer data for each patient audited on unit to Appendix C.9: Direct Nutrition Care Audit—Unit Summary.

Note: See Appendix D.7 for a completed example of this form.

APPENDIX C.9 DIRECT NUTRITION CARE AUDIT—UNIT SUMMARY

Unit _____ Auditor _____

Audit Dates _____ to _____ Nutritional Risk Level _____

Patient MR No.	Nutrition Assessment (1)	Monitoring and Reassessment (2)	Nutrition Education (3)	Food-Drug Interaction Counseling (4)	Case Management– Related Duties (5)	Other (6)	Total Nutrition Intervention Time (7)
Total time per activity (min)	A	B	C	D	E	F	Total intervention time (A + B + C + D + E + F)
Average time per activity (min)	A/G	B/G	C/G	D/G	E/G	F/G	Total no. of patients G

Min H
Average time per patient

Instructions (for Appendix C.9, p. 167):

1. Use this form to compile the data for all patients *at the same level of nutrition risk* on a unit for the audit period. *Complete separate forms for moderate-risk and high-risk patients.*

2. List the medical record (MR) numbers of all patients who received direct nutrition care in the left column of the form.

3. For each patient listed, enter the minutes spent in each activity in the columns numbered 1 through 6. In the column numbered 7, list total direct care time. Data for columns 1 through 7 come from Appendix C.8: Direct Nutrition Care Audit—Individual Patient form.

4. Determine the total amount of time (in minutes) spent on each activity by adding data in each column. Record the totals in the boxes on the next to the last row:
   • A = Total time for nutrition assessment
   • B = Total time for monitoring and reassessment
   • C = Total time for nutrition education
   • D = Total time for nutrient-drug interaction counseling
   • E = Total time for case management–related duties
   • F = Total time for other direct care activities (facility-specific)

5. Add the numbers in these boxes across to derive the total direct care time for the unit for patients at each level of nutrition risk. List this total in Box H.

6. Count the total number of patients receiving direct nutrition care during the audit period (ie, the total number of separate medical record numbers listed in the left column) and list this in Box G.

7. Transfer data for A, B, C, D, E, F, G, and H for all units audited to the appropriate boxes on Appendix C.10: Direct Care—Facility Summary.

Note: See Appendixes D.8–D.10 for completed examples of this form.

APPENDIX C.10 DIRECT NUTRITION CARE—FACILITY SUMMARY

Nutritional Risk Level ____

Unit	Nutrition Assessment (A) Minutes	Monitoring and Reassessment (B) Minutes	Nutrition Education (C) Minutes	Food-Drug Interaction Counseling (D) Minutes	Case Management–Related Duties (E) Minutes	Other (F) Minutes	No. of Patients in Unit Audit (G)	Total Nutrition Intervention Time (H) Minutes
Totals	Minutes I	Minutes J	Minutes K	Minutes L	Minutes M	Minutes N	Minutes O	Minutes P
Time per activity (min)	I/O	J/O	K/O	L/O	M/O	N/O		Average time per patient ____ at (1) nutritional risk level (P/O)

R-1

Instructions (for Appendix C.10, p. 169):

1. Use this form to compile data for all patients *at the same level of nutrition risk* for the entire facility during the audit period. *Complete separate forms for low-risk, moderate-risk, and high-risk patients.*
2. List the units in the far-left column on the form.
3. List the unit totals for each activity from Appendix C.9: Direct Nutrition Care Audit—Unit Summary (Boxes A, B, C, D and E, as well as Box F, if used).
4. List the total number of patients included in the audit by unit (Box G from Appendix C.9).
5. List the total amount of direct care time by unit (Box H from Appendix C.9).
6. Determine the total amount of time spent on each activity for the entire facility by adding data in each column. Record the totals in the boxes on the next-to-last row:
   - I = Total time for nutrition assessment
   - J = Total time for monitoring and reassessment
   - K = Total time for nutrition education
   - L = Total time for nutrient-drug interaction counseling
   - M = Total time for case management—related duties
   - N = Total time for other direct care activities (facility-specific)
7. For patients at each level of nutrition risk, add the numbers in Boxes I through N to derive the total direct care time (in minutes) for the unit. List this total in Box P.
8. Count the total number of patients receiving direct nutrition care during the audit period (column G) and list this in the Box O.
9. Calculate the per-activity averages for the facility by dividing the total time for each activity by the number listed in Box O.
10. Calculate the average direct care time per patient by dividing the number in Box P by the number in Box O. List this average time in Box R-1. Note: R-1 = Risk level 1 (ie, low risk). The process should be repeated to determine an average direct care time for each level of nutrition risk. For moderate risk, change box label to R-2; for high risk, change box label to R-3.
11. Transfer data for R-1, R-2, and R-3 to appropriate boxes in the Patient Care Staffing Estimates form (Appendix C.11).

Note: See Appendixes D.11–D.13 for completed examples of this form.

APPENDIX C.11   PATIENT CARE* STAFFING ESTIMATES

Activity	Time Factor (average time per patient)	No. of Patients/Year	Total Time Required/Year (minutes)	Total Time Required/Year (hours)
General nutrition care				
• Nutrition screening	S	Estimated no. of patients admitted to facility per year = ADM (use budgeted amount)	$S \times ADM$	
• Rescreening (if applicable)	T	P-1 × 52	M-1 × 52	
• Nutritional risk status evaluation (if applicable)	U	P-2 × 52	M-2 × 52	
• NPO and clear liquid monitoring (if applicable)	V	P-3 × 52	M-3 × 52	
Subtotal: general nutrition care			General care subtotal Minutes	General care subtotal minutes/60 = Hours
1:1 Nutrition intervention (select according to facility nutritional risk levels)				
• Nutritional risk level 1 (low risk)	R-1	$X^{\dagger} \times ADM$	$R\text{-}1 \times X \times ADM$	
• Nutritional risk level 2 (moderate risk)	R-2	$Y^{\dagger} \times ADM$	$R\text{-}2 \times Y \times ADM$	
• Nutritional risk level 3 (high risk)	R-3	$Z^{\dagger} \times ADM$	$R\text{-}3 \times Z \times ADM$	
Subtotal: direct care time			Direct care subtotal Minutes	Direct care subtotal minutes/60 = Hours
Total Patient Care Hours (add general care subtotal and direct care subtotal)			**Patient care total Minutes**	**Patient care total minutes/60 = Hours**
Total Patient Care FTEs‡				**Total patient care hours/2,080 = FTEs**

*Patient care = general nutrition care and direct nutrition care.

†Convert percentages to decimals.

‡Total patient care FTEs are added to FTEs for indirect and nonpatient care to calculate total FTEs. This number must be adjusted further to allow for vacation time, holidays, and other leave time.

Instructions:

General nutrition care:

1. List the total times for each of the unit-based activities from Appendix C.5 in the first four shaded boxes in the 5th column on the form.
2. Add the activity times to derive a subtotal of minutes. List this number in the General care subtotal—Minutes box.
3. Divide the subtotal of minutes by 60 to determine total hours in unit-based activities. List this number in the General care subtotal—Hours box.

Direct care:

1. Calculate the total time required per year for each activity listed by level of nutrition risk. Multiply the time factor for each risk level from Appendix C.3 (R-1, R-2, and R-3) by the percentage of patients admitted at that risk level (converted to a decimal) from Appendix C.3. Multiply that product by the number of patients admitted to the facility in 1 year from Appendix C.3. List this number in minutes in the shaded boxes for each risk level in the 5th column.

   For example: if time factor for R-1 = 45 minutes; 50 % of patients admitted are at low risk (X); and Admissions = 5, 000 per year, then $45 \times 0.5 \times 5000 = 112,500$ minutes

2. Add these 3 activity times to derive a subtotal of minutes for direct care. List the subtotal in the Direct care subtotal—Minutes box.
3. Divide the direct care subtotal by 60 to determine total hours in direct care activities for patients at all risk levels. List this number in the Direct care subtotal—Hours box.

Total patient care:

1. Add both subtotals to derive the total hours of time required for patient care activities for the facility for the year. List these numbers in the 6th row of the form (4th and 5th columns).
2. Divide the total number of hours by 2,080 hours to derive total full time equivalents (FTEs) required for patient care activity.

Note: See Appendix D.14 for a completed example of this form.

APPENDIX C.12 OUTPATIENT STAFFING PROJECTION

Diagnosis	Type 1 DM	Type 2 DM	GDM	HPL	CKD	WM*	Cancer*	Other Diagnoses	Totals
Estimated no. of 1:1 clients/year (1)									
1:1 MNT hours from GFP	5.0	3.5	3.75	2.5	4.0	4.0*	2.5*		
1:1 MNT hours (2)									
No. of MNT group sessions (3)									
Group MNT hours (3)									
Estimated additional client care hours (4)		Estimated indirect hours (5)		Vacation/ relief coverage hours (6)		Total hours (7)		FTEs (8)	

Abbreviations: ADA, American Dietetic Association; CKD, chronic kidney disease; DM, diabetes mellitus; FTEs, full-time equivalents; GDM, gestational diabetes mellitus; GFP, MNT Guide for Practice; HPL, hyperlipidemia; MNT, medical nutrition therapy; WM, weight management.

*MNT Guides for Practice are being developed. When published, check MNT Guide for Practice CD-ROMs for exact number of MNT hours.

Instructions:

1. Estimate the number of clients who will receive 1:1 MNT in the coming year, using past performance data and projected program goals.
2. Multiply the number of 1:1 clients by MNT hours from ADA MNT Guides for Practice and MNT Protocols. For diagnoses without protocols, multiply the number of 1:1 clients by estimated average MNT per client.
3. Estimate the number of MNT group sessions and hours of group MNT time.
4. Estimate the number of hours of additional client care—eg, additional MNT follow-up and prevention and wellness counseling (hours/month × 12).
5. Estimate the total indirect hours—eg, documentation, dietary analysis, meetings, program planning, marketing, and community presentations (hours/month × 12).
6. Estimate needed hours for relief coverage, if provided. Include vacation and professional and medical leaves.
7. Calculate total hours from all estimates, including 1:1 and group MNT hours.
8. Calculate FTEs required by dividing total hours by 2,080 hours (1 FTE).

Note: See Appendix D.15 for a completed example of this form.

APPENDIX C.13   STAFFING EVALUATION

Audit Period _____

Position	Calculated Needs (FTEs)	Actual/ Worked (FTEs)	Worked Variance (FTEs)	Worked Variance (%)	Budgeted FTEs	Budgeted Variance (FTEs)	Budgeted Variance (%)
Registered dietitians							
Dietetic technicians							
Totals							

Instructions:

1. List calculated full time equivalent (FTE) needs for dietitians and dietetic technicians in the column titled Calculated Needs. List actual/worked FTEs and budgeted FTEs for each position in the appropriate columns.

2. Substract actual/worked FTEs from calculated FTEs to determine Worked Variance FTEs. Divide actual/worked FTEs by calculated needs FTEs and multiply result by 100 to determine the Worked Variance percentage.

3. Substract budgeted FTEs from calculated FTEs to determine Budgeted Variance FTEs. Divide budgeted FTEs by calculated needs FTEs and multiply result by 100 to determine the Budgeted Variance percentage.

APPENDIX C.14   NUTRITION SERVICES STAFF PLAN AND SCHEDULE TEMPLATE

No. of Positions: RD _____   Dietetic Technician _____

FTEs: RD _____   Dietetic Technician _____

Month_____

	Sunday	Monday	Tuesday	Wednesday	Thursday	Friday	Saturday
RD coverage Units	Position	Position	Position	Position	Position	Position	Position
Totals • FTEs • No. of positions							
Dietetic technician coverage							
Units							
Totals • FTEs • No. of positions							

Instructions:

1. List all units that staff members cover in the far left column. List by position (ie, RDs together and dietetic technicians together). If desired, templates for RDs and dietetic technicians can be listed on separate pages.
2. Assign each position a number (eg, RD 1, RD 2, Tech 1, and Tech 2), and note assigned units.
3. List coverage for each day of the week by position numbers.
4. List the total number of positions and the total number of full-time equivalents (FTEs) working each day of the template.
5. The number of pages needed for the template will depend on the number of staff in the weekend rotation. For example, if six RDs work in the weekend rotation, the template will be six pages long.

Developing a Staffing Plan:
Completed Worksheets

APPENDIX D.1   COMPLETED ADMISSION NUTRITIONAL RISK AUDIT

Unit _____ 1North _____   Auditor _____ AB _____

Date	Total Number of Admissions	Low or No Risk	Moderate Risk	High Risk
10–6-04	3	2	1	0
10–7-04	4	1	2	1
10–8-04	3	0	2	1
10–9-04	3	1	1	1
10–10-04	4	2	1	1
10–11-04	2	1	1	0
10–12-04	1	0	0	1
Totals	20	7	8	5
%		35%	40%	25%

Instructions:

1. Complete an audit for a 7-day period. Staff on each unit should complete audits for the same 1-week interval. When possible, complete audits for 1-week intervals in each 3-month quarter of the year.
2. List the following data in the correct column, by date:
   - Total number of patients admitted to the unit.
   - Number of patients at each level of nutritional risk. Adjust the names and numbers of risk categories to correspond with facility procedures.
3. Add each column to obtain the total number of patients admitted to the unit for a 1-week period and the total numbers of patients in each nutritional risk category.
4. Calculate the percentage of patients in each risk category:
   (Total number of patients in risk category ÷ Total number of patients admitted to unit during 1-week interval) × 100.

Note: The template for this form is found in Appendix C.1.

APPENDIX D.2   COMPLETED ADMISSION NUTRITIONAL RISK SUMMARY

Dates of Audit _____*10-6-04*_____ to _____*10-12-04*_____

Unit	Total Number of Admissions	Low or No Risk	Moderate Risk	High Risk
1 North	20	7	8	5
2 North*	22	11	5	6
3 North*	16	7	4	5
Totals	58	25	17	16
%		43% **X**	29% **Y**	28% **Z**

*Audit data not shown.

Instructions:

1. List the total numbers of admissions and patients in each category of nutritional risk for each unit.
2. Add each column to obtain the total number of patients admitted to all units for the 1-week period and the total numbers of patients in each nutritional risk category.
3. Calculate the percentage of patients in each risk category for the entire facility:
   (Total number of patients in risk category ÷ Total number of patients admitted to facility during 1-week interval) × 100.
   X = percentage of low-risk patients; Y = percentage of moderate-risk patients; and Z = percentage of high-risk patients.
4. Transfer calculated percentages for X, Y, and Z to two locations in Appendix C.11: Patient Care Staffing Estimates.

Note: The template for this form is found in Appendix C.2.

APPENDIX D.3   COMPLETED GENERAL NUTRITION CARE TIME AUDIT

Unit _1North_   Auditor _AB_   Audit Dates _10-6-04_ to _10-12-04_

Patient MR No.	Nutrition Screening			Patient MR No.	Rescreening			Patient MR No.	Nutritional Risk Status Evaluation		
	Start	Stop	Minutes		Start	Stop	Minutes		Start	Stop	Minutes
101	7:15	7:25	10	101	9:01	9:12	11				
102	7:25	7:36	11	102	9:12	9:22	10	102	9:22	9:43	21
103	7:38	7:45	7					103	7:45	7:55	10
104	7:05	7:14	9					104	7:14	7:29	15
105	7:30	7:41	11	105	9:00	9:14	14				
106	7:41	7:50	9					106	7:50	8:05	15
107	8:05	8:16	11					107	8:16	8:31	15
108	7:15	7:29	14					108	7:29	7:41	12
109	7:42	7:52	10					109	7:52	8:04	12
110	8:04	8:13	9					110	8:13	8:27	14
111	7:10	7:21	11					111	7:21	7:36	15
112	7:38	7:49	11					112	7:49	8:02	13
113	8:04	8:15	11	113	9:02	9:16	14	113	9:16	9:31	15
114	7:15	7:26	11					114	7:26	7:41	15
115	7:41	7:54	13					115	7:54	8:09	15
116	8:09	8:20	11								
117	8:20	8:32	12	117	9:15	9:26	11				
118	7:15	7:26	11	118	9:07	9:19	12	118	9:19	9:31	12
119	7:26	7:37	11					119	7:37	7:55	18
120	7:10	7:21	11					120	7:21	7:37	16
Total no.	20	Total time	214 min	Total no.	6	Total time	72 min	Total no.	16	Total time	233 min
		Average	10.7 min			Average	12 min			Average	14.6 min

Unit _1North_   **Auditor** _AB_   **Audit Dates** _10-6-04_ to _10-12-04_

Patient MR No.	NPO and Clear Liquid Monitoring			Patient MR No.	_____			Patient MR No.	_____		
	Start	Stop	Minutes		Start	Stop	Minutes		Start	Stop	Minutes
104	1:15	1:21	6								
107	1:25	1:35	10								
112	1:02	1:13	11								
113	1:15	1:26	11								
Total no.	4	Total time	38 min	Total no.		Total time		Total no.		Total time	
		Average	9.5 min			Average				Average	

Instructions:

1. Choose a week (7 days) when all staff are working (ie, no vacations or other leave are scheduled). Each staff member should complete his/her own audit form.
2. Include data for weekend coverage (ie, staff working the weekend should record data for these days, as well as other days worked during the week). Columns have been included for other unit-based activities that are not listed on the form but are completed by clinical nutrition staff at the facility.
3. Record the medical record number (MR No.) for each patient for whom nutrition care is provided during the audit period.

4. List the start and stop times for each of the listed activities completed for each patient. For example: Nutrition screening started at 10:00 a.m. and stopped at 10:12 a.m.

5. Calculate and list the minutes spent on each activity for each patient.

6. Record the total number of patients for whom each activity was completed during the audit period in the shaded "Total no." boxes on the next-to-last line of the form.

7. Add the total number of minutes spent in each activity during the audit period and list this in the shaded "Total time" boxes on the next-to-last line of the form.

8. Calculate the average time spent on each activity by dividing the total number of minutes spent on the activity by the number of patients for that activity. Record the average times for each activity in the shaded boxes on the last line of the form. Transfer data for all audited units to Appendix C.5: General Nutrition Care Time Audit Summary.

Note: The template for this form in found in Appendix C.4.

APPENDIX D.4   COMPLETED GENERAL NUTRITION CARE TIME AUDIT SUMMARY

Audit Dates ___10-6-04___ to ___10-12-04___ (7-day interval)

Unit	Nutrition Screening		Rescreening		Nutritional Risk Status Evaluation		NPO and Clear Liquid Monitoring		(Add Other Activities As Needed)	
	Minutes	Patients	Minutes	Patients	Minutes	Patients	Minutes	Patients	Minutes	Patients
1 North	214	20	72	6	233	16	38	4		
2 North*	232	22	131	10	198	14	92	8		
3 North*	185	16	60	5	171	12	40	3		
Total	Minutes 631	Patients 58	Minutes (M-1) 263	Patients (P-1) 21	Minutes (M-2) 602	Patients (P-2) 42	Minutes (M-3) 170	Patients (P-3) 15		
Per-patient averages	10.9 min S		12.5 min T		14.3 min U		11.3 min V			
Annual time estimates	S × No. of admits 10.9 × 3,000 = 32,700 min		M-1 × 52 13,676 min		M-2 × 52 31,304 min		M-3 × 52 8,840 min			

* Audit data not shown

Instructions (for Appendix D.4, p. 183):

1. List the units included in the audit in the shaded column on the left of the form.
2. List the total number of minutes spent in each activity for each unit audited from Appendix C.4: General Nutrition Care Time Audit. List the total number of patients for each activity by unit from Appendix C.4. Include data from all staff who worked on each unit during the audit period, including weekends.
3. Add the unit totals to get the facility total of number of minutes for each activity for the audit period (1 week) and the total number of patients for each activity for the audit period.
4. The results for rescreening, nutrition risk status evaluation, and NPO/clear liquid monitoring are assigned codes:
   - M-1 for rescreening time
   - M-2 for nutrition risk status evaluation time
   - M-3 for NPO/clear liquid monitoring time
   - P-1 for rescreening patients
   - P-2 for nutrition risk status evaluation patients
   - P-3 for NPO/clear liquid monitoring patients).
5. Calculate facility's per-patient averages for each activity by dividing total time spent per activity during the audit period by the total number of patients for each activity. A letter code has been assigned to each average:
   - S = average time per nutrition screen
   - T = average time rescreening
   - U = average time per nutrition risk status evaluation
   - V = average time per NPO/clear liquid monitoring.
6. Estimate facility's total annual time for each activity as follows:
   - Nutrition screening = S multiplied by the number of patients admitted to the facility per year. (The number of admissions is obtained from facility reports.) Logic: each patient admitted to the facility must have a nutrition screening.
   - Rescreening = M-1 mulitiplied by 52. Logic: not all patients will need to be rescreened. Assuming that the weekly average time calculated from the audit is representative of a typical week, this number is multiplied by 52 to derive an annual estimate.
   - Nutrition risk evaluation = M-2 multiplied by 52. Assuming that the weekly average time calculated from the audit is representative of a typical week, this number is multiplied by 52 to derive an annual estimate.
   - NPO/clear liquid monitoring = M-3 multiplied by 52. Assuming that the weekly average time calculated from the audit is representative of a typical week, this number is multiplied by 52 to derive an annual estimate.
7. Transfer the annual time estimates for each unit-based activity to the Patient Care Staffing Estimates form in Appendix C.11.

Note: The template for this form is found in Appendix C.5.

APPENDIX D.5　COMPLETED ACTIVITY TIME AUDIT—INDIRECT AND NONPATIENT CARE

Unit _1 North_ 　　Auditor _LM (RD)_ 　　Audit Dates _10-60-04_ to _10-12-04*_

Date	Daily Organizational Activities			Team Rounds			Group Patient Education		
	Start	Stop	Minutes	Start	Stop	Minutes	Start	Stop	Minutes
10-6-04	7:00	7:20	20	7:30	8:30	60			
10-6-04	3:15	3:45	30						
10-7-04	7:00	7:15	15						
10-7-04	3:10	3:30	20						
10-8-04	7:00	7:20	20	7:30	8:30	60			
10-8-04	3:15	3:30	15						
10-9-04	7:00	7:25	25				1:30	2:30	60
10-9-04	3:15	3:30	15						
10-10-04	7:00	7:15	15	7:30	8:30	60			
10-10-04	3:15	3:35	20						
		Total time	195 min		Total time	180 min		Total time	60 min

*LM collected data for the 5 days worked during the 7-day interval from 10-6-04 to 10-12-04.

(*continues*)

APPENDIX D.5   (*continued*)

Unit __1 North__   Auditor __LM (RD)__   Audit Dates __10-60-04__ to __10-12-04*__

Date	Indirect Care Activities			Student Training			Nonpatient Care		
	Start	Stop	Minutes	Start	Stop	Minutes	Start	Stop	Minutes
10–6-04									
10–7-04	1:00	2:00	60						
10–8-04				10:00	11:30	90			
10–9-04							10:00	11:00	60
10–10-04									
		Total time	60 min		Total time	90 min		Total time	60 min

*LM collected data for the 5 days worked during the 7-day interval from 10-6-04 to 10-12-04.

Instructions:

1. This form is used to determine the amount of time spent on indirect care and non–patient care activities for a 7-day interval. Each member of the staff should track his/her own information using a separate form.
2. For each day of the audit, record start and stop times for each type of activity listed. Use the information below to determine how to categorize activity types. List activities as many times as they take place (ie, types of activities may be listed more than once per day).
3. Calculate the number of minutes spent on each activity and list this in the column headed "Minutes."
4. Calculate the total minutes for each type of activity by adding the minutes for each activity. List in the unshaded box in the last row on the form.
5. Transfer the data for each staff member participating in the audit to Appendix C.7: Activity Time Audit Summary—Indirect and Nonpatient Care.

Indirect Care Activities:

- Project planning and work time
- Meetings
- Providing and receiving job-related training, including time spent planning training and creating handouts
- Community programs, classes, and support groups
- Performance improvement projects and activities
- Outcomes data collection and related activities
- Research
- Food service activities

Non–Patient Care Time

- Travel time from one work area to another
- Personal breaks
- Delays

Daily Organizational Activities:

- Checking patient lists and generating computer reports
- Planning workload
- Discussions about workload and assignments with other clinical nutrition staff, including providing updates related to days off, weekend coverage, and/or patient transfers
- Updating computer or patient files related to workload
- Email and correspondence
- Telephone calls unrelated to patient care. (calls that are not case management activities)

Team Rounds:

- Bedside rounds and other health care team rounds
- Care planning meetings and conferences
- Discharge planning meetings

Student Training:

- Time spent preparing for, training, providing oversight to, and evaluating dietetic interns and/or students
- Classes taught to dietetic interns, including planning and preparation time
- Classes and programs for other students, including planning and preparation time

Group Patient Care Education:

- Preparation for, conducting, and documenting group nutrition education programs for patients and/or family members

Note: The template for this form is found in Appendix C.6.

APPENDIX D.6   COMPLETED ACTIVITY TIME AUDIT SUMMARY—INDIRECT AND NONPATIENT CARE

Audit Dates   10-6-04   **to**   10-12-04   (7-day interval)*

Staff Name	Daily Organizational Activities	Team Rounds	Group Patient Education	Indirect Care Activities	Student Training	Nonpatient Care
LM	195	180	60	60	90	60
RS†	150	30	0	60	0	45
TW†	160	0	0	120	0	60
Subtotal	505 Minutes	210 Minutes	60 Minutes	240 Minutes	90 Minutes	165 Minutes
Divide minutes by 60	8.4 Hours	3.5 Hours	1.0 Hours	4.0 Hours	1.5 Hours	2.75 Hours
Adjusted time requirements	Hours	Hours	Hours	Hours	Hours	Hours
Total time/week: Add hours for each type of activity.	Total time/week: 21.15 Hours					
	Total time/year: Multiply total time/week by 52.	1,100 Hours 0.53 FTEs				

*Each RD collected data for the 5 days worked during the interval from 10–6-04 to 10–12-04. (LM and RS worked 10–6-04 to 10–10-04. TW worked 10–08-04 to 10–12-04.)

†Audit data not shown.

Instructions:

1. In the left column, list the names of all staff who participated in the audit.
2. Record the number of minutes spent by each staff member on each type of activity, from Appendix C.6: Activity Time Audit-Indirect and Non–Patient Care.
3. Add the minutes in each column to obtain a total number of minutes spent by all staff for each activity. Record the total minutes for each type of activity in the Subtotal row of the form.
4. Convert minutes to hours (divide number of minutes by 60).
5. Make adjustments in time requirements as needed. Refer to Notes below. If no adjustments are needed, the numbers in this row are the same as those on the prior row.
6. Calculate the total hours required per week by adding the number of hours in each box in the Adjusted Time Requirements row. List this total in the second box from the left in the last row on the form.
7. Multiply this number (ie, the total derived in step 6) by 52 to calculate the yearly total for indirect care and non–patient care activities. List in the farthest right unshaded box on the last row of the form.
8. Divide the yearly total in hours by 2,080 to derive the number of FTEs required. List in the same box.

Notes:

*   When determining weekly time totals for each activity, evaluate factors that might increase or decrease weekly requirement and make adjustments in totals as appropriate. For example, if dietetic interns are present for three fourths of the year, the required weekly time would need to be adjusted to reflect this. Because of staff involvement in other types of student training, it may not be accurate to adjust the time per week to three fourths of the calculated amount. However, a reduction below the calculated amount will be indicated.
*   In lieu of doing an audit, staff can estimate the time spent in each activity. These data can be recorded on the Activity Time Audit Summary, and a final time requirement can be estimated as described above (ie, total time for each activity is determined by adding estimates for each activity for all staff and making any adjustments to reflect variation based on schedules, etc).

Note: The template for this form is found in Appendix C.7.

Unit ___1North___   Patient MR No. ___104___   Nutritional Risk Level ___High___

Auditor ___LM___   Audit Dates ___10-1-04___ to ___10-31-04___

Date Admit date:	Nutrition Assessment			Monitoring and Reassessment			Nutrition Education			Nutrition-Drug Interaction Counseling			Case Management—Related Duties			Other		
	Start	Stop	Min	Start	Stop	Min	Start	Stop	Min	Start	Stop	Min	Start	Stop	Min	Start	Stop	Min
10-6-04																		
10-7-04	7:45	8:30	45															
10-10-04				10:00	10:20	20												
10-14-04				9:45	10:10	25	11:00	11:20	20	10:20	10:35	15						
Total activity time (min)	45(1)			45(2)			20(3)			15(4)			0(5)			0(6)		
Total intervention (min) (Add 1–6)	125(7)																	

Instructions:

1. This form is used to determine the amount of time spent in direct care.
2. One form needs to be completed for each patient receiving direct nutrition care during the audit period. For each patient, list at the top of the form the unit, patient's medical record number, and nutrition risk level.
3. Record activities by date. List the start and stop times for each activity performed. Calculate the number of minutes spent in each activity and record for each activity in the shaded columns headed "Min."
4. Add the minutes for each activity and record in the second-to-last row on the form.
   - Box 1 = Total time for nutrition assessment
   - Box 2 = Total time for monitoring and reassessment
   - Box 3 = Total time for nutrition education
   - Box 4 = Total time for nutrient-drug interaction counseling
   - Box 5 = Total time for case management-related duties
   - Box 6 = Total time for other direct care activities (facility-specific)
5. Determine total direct care time for each patient by adding the totals for all activities. List this total in Box 7. Transfer data for each patient audited on unit to Appendix C.9: Direct Nutrition Care Audit—Unit Summary.

Note: The template for this form is found in Appendix C.8.

APPENDIX D.8 COMPLETED DIRECT NUTRITION CARE AUDIT—UNIT SUMMARY: LOW RISK

Unit __1North__   Auditor __AB__

Audit Dates __10-1-04__ to __10-31-04__   Nutritional Risk Level __LowRisk—Week 2 Admissions Listed__

Patient MR No.	Nutrition Assessment (1)	Monitoring and Reassessment (2)	Nutrition Education (3)	Food-Drug Interaction Counseling (4)	Case Management–Related Duties (5)	Other (6)	Total Nutrition Intervention Time (7)
101	0	0	15	0	0	10	25
102	0	0	0	15	0	0	15
105	0	0	0	15	0	5	20
113	0	0	20	0	0	0	20
116	0	0	25	0	0	0	25
117	0	0	10	0	0	10	20
118	0	0	0	0	0	15	15
Total time per activity (min)	0 — A	0 — B	308 — C	132 — D	0 — E	154 — F	Total intervention time (A + B + C + D + E + F) 594 Min — H
Average time per activity (min)	0 — A/G	0 — B/G	10 — C/G	4 — D/G	0 — E/G	5 — F/G	Total no. of patients 31 — G
							Average time per patient 19min

*Data from *all* October low-risk admissions on 1 North were combined to derive totals.

Instructions:

1. Use this form to compile the data for all patients *at the same level of nutrition risk* on a unit for the audit period. *Complete separate forms for moderate-risk and high-risk patients.*

2. List the medical record (MR) numbers of all patients who received direct nutrition care in the left column of the form.

3. For each patient listed, enter the minutes spent in each activity in the columns numbered 1 through 6. In the column numbered 7, list total direct care time. Data for columns 1 through 7 come from Appendix C.8: Direct Nutrition Care Audit—Individual Patient form.

4. Determine the total amount of time (in minutes) spent on each activity by adding data in each column. Record the totals in the boxes on the next to the last row:
   - A = Total time for nutrition assessment
   - B = Total time for monitoring and reassessment
   - C = Total time for nutrition education
   - D = Total time for nutrient-drug interaction counseling
   - E = Total time for case management—related duties
   - F = Total time for other direct care activities (facility-specific)

5. Add the numbers in these boxes across to derive the total direct care time for the unit for patients at each level of nutrition risk. List this total in Box H.

6. Count the total number of patients receiving direct nutrition care during the audit period (ie, the total number of separate medical record numbers listed in the left column) and list this in Box G.

7. Transfer data for A, B, C, D, E, F, G, and H for all units audited to the appropriate boxes on Appendix C.10: Direct Care—Facility Summary.

Note: The template for this form is found in Appendix C.9.

APPENDIX D.9 COMPLETED DIRECT NUTRITION CARE AUDIT—UNIT SUMMARY: MODERATE RISK

Unit ___1North___   Auditor ___AB___

Audit Dates ___10-1-04___ to ___10-31-04___ Nutritional Risk Level ___Moderate Risk—Week 2 Admissions Listed___

Patient MR No.	Nutrition Assessment (1)	Monitoring and Reassessment (2)	Nutrition Education (3)	Food-Drug Interaction Counseling (4)	Case Management–Related Duties (5)	Other (6)	Total Nutrition Intervention Time (7)
103	35	15	10	0	0	0	50
106	25	20	15	10	0	10	80
107	30	10	15	0	0	0	55
109	25	20	0	10	0	0	55
110	30	20	15	0	0	0	65
112	30	15	10	0	0	10	65
115	35	10	0	10	0	0	55
119	30	15	15	0	0	0	60
Total time per activity (min)	1,056 A	550 B	352 C	132 D	0 E	88 F	2,178 Min H — Total intervention time (A + B + C + D + E + F)
Average time per activity (min)	30 A/G	16 B/G	10 C/G	4 D/G	0 E/G	3 F/G	35 G — Total no. of patients; Average time per patient 62 min

*Data from *all* October moderate-risk admissions on 1 North were combined to derive totals.

Instructions:

1. Use this form to compile the data for all patients *at the same level of nutrition risk* on a unit for the audit period. *Complete separate forms for moderate-risk and high-risk patients.*
2. List the medical record (MR) numbers of all patients who received direct nutrition care in the left column of the form.
3. For each patient listed, enter the minutes spent in each activity in the columns numbered 1 through 6. In the column numbered 7, list total direct care time. Data for columns 1 through 7 come from Appendix C.8: Direct Nutrition Care Audit—Individual Patient form.
4. Determine the total amount of time (in minutes) spent on each activity by adding data in each column. Record the totals in the boxes on the next to the last row:
   - A = Total time for nutrition assessment
   - B = Total time for monitoring and reassessment
   - C = Total time for nutrition education
   - D = Total time for nutrient-drug interaction counseling
   - E = Total time for case management—related duties
   - F = Total time for other direct care activities (facility-specific)
5. Add the numbers in these boxes across to derive the total direct care time for the unit for patients at each level of nutrition risk. List this total in Box H.
6. Count the total number of patients receiving direct nutrition care during the audit period (ie, the total number of separate medical record numbers listed in the left column) and list this in Box G.
7. Transfer data for A, B, C, D, E, F, G, and H for all units audited to the appropriate boxes on Appendix C.10: Direct Care—Facility Summary.

Note: The template for this form is found in Appendix C.9.

APPENDIX D.10 COMPLETED DIRECT NUTRITION CARE AUDIT—UNIT SUMMARY: MODERATE RISK

Unit ___1North___ Auditor ___LM___

Audit Dates ___10-1-04___ to ___10-31-04___ Nutritional Risk Level ___High Risk—Week 2 Admissions Listed___

Patient MR No.	Nutrition Assessment (1)	Monitoring and Reassessment (2)	Nutrition Education (3)	Food-Drug Interaction Counseling (4)	Case Management–Related Duties (5)	Other (6)	Total Nutrition Intervention Time (7)
104	45	45	20	0	15	0	125
108	40	60	10	0	0	20	130
111	42	40	0	15	0	0	97
114	46	80	20	0	15	20	181
120	45	45	15	0	0	0	105
Total time per activity (min)	959 A	1.188 B	286 C	66 D	132 E	176 F	Total intervention time (A+B+C+D+E+F) 2,807 Min H
Average time per activity (min)	44 A/G	54 B/G	13 C/G	3 D/G	6 E/G	8 F/G	Total no. of patients 22 G / Average time per patient 128 min

*Data from *all* October high-risk admissions on 1 North were combined to derive totals.

Instructions:

1. Use this form to compile the data for all patients *at the same level of nutrition risk* on a unit for the audit period. *Complete separate forms for moderate-risk and high-risk patients.*

2. List the medical record (MR) numbers of all patients who received direct nutrition care in the left column of the form.

3. For each patient listed, enter the minutes spent in each activity in the columns numbered 1 through 6. In the column numbered 7, list total direct care time. Data for columns 1 through 7 come from Appendix C.8: Direct Nutrition Care Audit—Individual Patient form.

4. Determine the total amount of time (in minutes) spent on each activity by adding data in each column. Record the totals in the boxes on the next to the last row:
   - A = Total time for nutrition assessment
   - B = Total time for monitoring and reassessment
   - C = Total time for nutrition education
   - D = Total time for nutrient-drug interaction counseling
   - E = Total time for case management—related duties
   - F = Total time for other direct care activities (facility-specific)

5. Add the numbers in these boxes across to derive the total direct care time for the unit for patients at each level of nutrition risk. List this total in Box H.

6. Count the total number of patients receiving direct nutrition care during the audit period (ie, the total number of separate medical record numbers listed in the left column) and list this in Box G.

7. Transfer data for A, B, C, D, E, F, G, and H for all units audited to the appropriate boxes on Appendix C.10: Direct Care—Facility Summary.

Note: The template for this form is found in Appendix C.9.

APPENDIX D.11 COMPLETED DIRECT NUTRITION CARE—FACILITY SUMMARY: LOW RISK

Nutritional Risk Level __Low__

Unit	Nutrition Assessment (A) Minutes	Monitoring and Reassessment (B) Minutes	Nutrition Education (C) Minutes	Food-Drug Interaction Counseling (D) Minutes	Case Management—Related Duties (E) Minutes	Other (F) Minutes	No. of Patients in Unit Audit (G)	Total Nutrition Intervention Time (H) Minutes
1North	0	0	308	132	0	154	31	594
2North	0	0	250	150	0	170	36	570
3North	0	0	275	120	0	145	29	540
Totals	0 Minutes I	0 Minutes J	833 Minutes K	402 Minutes L	0 Minutes M	469 Minutes N	96 Minutes O	1,704 Minutes P
Time per activity (min)	0 I/O	0 J/O	9 K/O	4 L/O	0 M/O	5 N/O		Average time per patient 18 min (1) at nutritional risk level (P/O) R-1

Instructions:

1. Use this form to compile data for all patients *at the same level of nutrition risk* for the entire facility during the audit period. *Complete separate forms for low-risk, moderate-risk, and high-risk patients.*

2. List the units in the far-left column on the form.

3. List the unit totals for each activity from Appendix C.9: Direct Nutrition Care Audit—Unit Summary (Boxes A, B, C, D and E, as well as Box F, if used).

4. List the total number of patients included in the audit by unit (Box G from Appendix C.9).

5. List the total amount of direct care time by unit (Box H from Appendix C.9).

6. Determine the total amount of time spent on each activity for the entire facility by adding data in each column. Record the totals in the boxes on the next-to-last row:
   - I = Total time for nutrition assessment
   - J = Total time for monitoring and reassessment
   - K = Total time for nutrition education
   - L = Total time for nutrient-drug interaction counseling
   - M = Total time for case management–related duties
   - N = Total time for other direct care activities (facility-specific)

7. For patients at each level of nutrition risk, add the numbers in Boxes I through N to derive the total direct care time (in minutes) for the unit. List this total in Box P.

8. Count the total number of patients receiving direct nutrition care during the audit period (column G) and list this in the Box O.

9. Calculate the per-activity averages for the facility by dividing the total time for each activity by the number listed in Box O.

10. Calculate the average direct care time per patient by dividing the number in Box P by the number in Box O. List this average time in Box R-1. Note: R-1 = Risk level 1 (ie, low risk). The process should be repeated to determine an average direct care time for each level of nutrition risk. For moderate risk, change box label to R-2; for high risk, change box label to R-3.

11. Transfer data for R-1, R-2, and R-3 to appropriate boxes in the Patient Care Staffing Estimates form (Appendix C.11).

Note: The template for this form is found in Appendix C.10.

APPENDIX D.12   COMPLETED DIRECT NUTRITION CARE—FACILITY SUMMARY: MODERATE RISK

Nutritional Risk Level   _Moderate_

Unit	Nutrition Assessment (A) Minutes	Monitoring and Reassessment (B) Minutes	Nutrition Education (C) Minutes	Food-Drug Interaction Counseling (D) Minutes	Case Management—Related Duties (E) Minutes	Other (F) Minutes	No. of Patients in Unit Audit (G)	Total Nutrition Intervention Time (H) Minutes
1North	1,056	550	352	132	0	88	35	2,178
2North	998	530	401	114	0	101	40	2,144
3North	1,022	560	375	151	0	72	33	2,179
Totals	3,076 Minutes I	1,145 Minutes J	1,128 Minutes K	397 Minutes L	0 Minutes M	261 Minutes N	108 Minutes O	6,501 Minutes P
Time per activity (min)	29 I/O	11 J/O	10 K/O	4 L/O	0 M/O	2 N/O		Average time per patient _60 min_ (1) at nutritional risk level (P/O)

R-2

Instructions:

1. Use this form to compile data for all patients *at the same level of nutrition risk* for the entire facility during the audit period. *Complete separate forms forlow-risk, moderate-risk, and high-risk patients.*
2. List the units in the far-left column on the form.
3. List the unit totals for each activity from Appendix C.9: Direct Nutrition Care Audit—Unit Summary (Boxes A, B, C, D and E, as well as Box F, if used).
4. List the total number of patients included in the audit by unit (Box G from Appendix C.9).
5. List the total amount of direct care time by unit (Box H from Appendix C.9).
6. Determine the total amount of time spent on each activity for the entire facility by adding data in each column. Record the totals in the boxes on the next-to-last row:
    *   I = Total time for nutrition assessment
    *   J = Total time for monitoring and reassessment
    *   K = Total time for nutrition education
    *   L = Total time for nutrient-drug interaction counseling
    *   M = Total time for case management–related duties
    *   N = Total time for other direct care activities (facility-specific)
7. For patients at each level of nutrition risk, add the numbers in Boxes I through N to derive the total direct care time (in minutes) for the unit. List this total in Box P.
8. Count the total number of patients receiving direct nutrition care during the audit period (column G) and list this in the Box O.
9. Calculate the per-activity averages for the facility by dividing the total time for each activity by the number listed in Box O.
10. Calculate the average direct care time per patient by dividing the number in Box P by the number in Box O. List this average time in Box R-1. Note: R-1 = Risk level 1 (ie, low risk). The process should be repeated to determine an average direct care time for each level of nutrition risk. For moderate risk, change box label to R-2; for high risk, change box label to R-3.
11. Transfer data for R-1, R-2, and R-3 to appropriate boxes in the Patient Care Staffing Estimates form (Appendix C.11).

Note: The template for this form is found in Appendix C.10.

APPENDIX D.13   COMPLETED DIRECT NUTRITION CARE—FACILITY SUMMARY: HIGH RISK

Nutritional Risk Level __High__

Unit	Nutrition Assessment (A) Minutes	Monitoring and Reassessment (B) Minutes	Nutrition Education (C) Minutes	Food-Drug Interaction Counseling (D) Minutes	Case Management—Related Duties (E) Minutes	Other (F) Minutes	No. of Patients in Unit Audit (G)	Total Nutrition Intervention Time (H) Minutes
1 North	959	1,188	286	66	132	176	22	2,807
2 North	1,022	1,225	301	72	100	150	19	2,870
3 North	1,015	1,170	294	61	125	160	24	2,825
Totals	2,996 Minutes I	3,583 Minutes J	881 Minutes K	199 Minutes L	357 Minutes M	486 Minutes N	65 Patients O	8,502 Minutes P
Time per activity (min)	46 I/O	55 J/O	14 K/O	3 L/O	5 M/O	8 N/O		Average time per patient 131min (1) at nutritional risk level (P/O)

R-3

Instructions:

1. Use this form to compile data for all patients *at the same level of nutrition risk* for the entire facility during the audit period. *Complete separate forms forlow-risk, moderate-risk, and high-risk patients.*
2. List the units in the far-left column on the form.
3. List the unit totals for each activity from Appendix C.9: Direct Nutrition Care Audit—Unit Summary (Boxes A, B, C, D and E, as well as Box F, if used).
4. List the total number of patients included in the audit by unit (Box G from Appendix C.9).
5. List the total amount of direct care time by unit (Box H from Appendix C.9).
6. Determine the total amount of time spent on each activity for the entire facility by adding data in each column. Record the totals in the boxes on the next-to-last row:
   - I = Total time for nutrition assessment
   - J = Total time for monitoring and reassessment
   - K = Total time for nutrition education
   - L = Total time for nutrient-drug interaction counseling
   - M = Total time for case management–related duties
   - N = Total time for other direct care activities (facility-specific)
7. For patients at each level of nutrition risk, add the numbers in Boxes I through N to derive the total direct care time (in minutes) for the unit. List this total in Box P.
8. Count the total number of patients receiving direct nutrition care during the audit period (column G) and list this in the Box O.
9. Calculate the per-activity averages for the facility by dividing the total time for each activity by the number listed in Box O.
10. Calculate the average direct care time per patient by dividing the number in Box P by the number in Box O. List this average time in Box R-1. Note: R-1 = Risk level 1 (ie, low risk). The process should be repeated to determine an average direct care time for each level of nutrition risk. For moderate risk, change box label to R-2; for high risk, change box label to R-3.
11. Transfer data for R-1, R-2, and R-3 to appropriate boxes in the Patient Care Staffing Estimates form (Appendix C.11).

Note: The template for this form is found in Appendix C.10.

APPENDIX D.14   COMPLETED PATIENT CARE* STAFFING ESTIMATES

Activity	Time Factor (average time per patient)	No. of Patients/Year	Total Time Required/Year (minutes)	Total Time Required/Year (hours)
General nutrition care				
• Nutrition screening	S	Estimated no. of patients admitted to facility per year = ADM (use budgeted amount)	S × ADM	32,700 min = 545 hours
• Rescreening (if applicable)	T	P-1 × 52	M-1 × 52	13,676 min = 228 hours
• Nutritional risk status evaluation (if applicable)	U	P-2 × 52	M-2 × 52	31,304 min = 522 hours
• NPO and clear liquid monitoring (if applicable)	V	P-3 × 52	M-3 × 52	8,840 min = 147 hours
Subtotal: general nutrition care			General care subtotal 86,520 Minutes	General care subtotal minutes/60 1,442 Hours
1:1 Nutrition intervention (select according to facility nutritional risk levels)				
• Nutritional risk level 1 (low risk)	R-1	X† × ADM	R-1 × X × ADM 18 × 0.43 × 3,000	23,200 min = 387 hours
• Nutritional risk level 2 (moderate risk)	R-2	Y† × ADM	R-2 × Y × ADM 60 × 0.29 × 3,000	52,200 min = 870 hours
• Nutritional risk level 3 (high risk)	R-3	Z† × ADM	R-3 × Z × ADM 131 × 0.28 × 3,000	110,040 min = 1,834 hours
Subtotal: direct care time			Direct care subtotal 185,440 Minutes	Direct care subtotal minutes/60 = 3,091 Hours
Total Patient Care Hours (add general care subtotal and direct care subtotal)			**Patient care total** 185,440 + 86,520 **Minutes**	**Patient care total minutes/60 =** 4,533 **Hours**
Total Patient Care FTEs‡				**Total patient care hours/2,080 =** 2.2 **FTEs**

*Patient care = general nutrition care and direct nutrition care.

†Convert percentages to decimals.

‡Total patient care FTEs are added to FTEs for indirect and nonpatient care to calculate total FTEs. This number must be adjusted further to allow for vacation time, holidays, and other leave time.

Instructions:

General nutrition care:

1. List the total times for each of the unit-based activities from Appendix C.5 in the first four shaded boxes in the 5th column on the form.
2. Add the activity times to derive a subtotal of minutes. List this number in the General care subtotal—Minutes box.
3. Divide the subtotal of minutes by 60 to determine total hours in unit-based activities. List this number in the General care subtotal—Hours box.

Direct care:

1. Calculate the total time required per year for each activity listed by level of nutrition risk. Multiply the time factor for each risk level from Appendix C.3 (R-1, R-2, and R-3) by the percentage of patients admitted at that risk level (converted to a decimal) from Appendix C.3. Multiply that product by the number of patients admitted to the facility in 1 year from Appendix C.3. List this number in minutes in the shaded boxes for each risk level in the 5th column.

   For example: if time factor for R-1 = 45 minutes; 50 % of patients admitted are at low risk (X); and Admissions = 5, 000 per year, then $45 \times 0.5 \times 5000 = 112{,}500$ minutes
2. Add these 3 activity times to derive a subtotal of minutes for direct care. List the subtotal in the Direct care subtotal—Minutes box.
3. Divide the direct care subtotal by 60 to determine total hours in direct care activities for patients at all risk levels. List this number in the Direct care subtotal—Hours box.

Total patient care:

1. Add both subtotals to derive the total hours of time required for patient care activities for the facility for the year. List these numbers in the 6th row of the form (4th and 5th columns).
2. Divide the total number of hours by 2,080 hours to derive total full time equivalents (FTEs) required for patient care activity.

Note: The template for this form is found in Appendix C.11.

APPENDIX D.15   COMPLETED OUTPATIENT STAFFING PROJECTION

Diagnosis	Type 1 DM	Type 2 DM	GDM	HPL	CKD	WM*	Cancer*	Other Diagnoses	Totals
Estimated no. of 1:1 clients/year (1)	300	1,000	150	500	150	1,000	500	320	4,570 patients
1:1 MNT hours from GFP	5.0	3.5	3.75	2.5	4.0	4.0*	2.5*		
1:1 MNT hours (2)	1,500	2,625	563	1,250	600	4,000	1,250	640	12,428 hours
No. of MNT group sessions (3)		4-week session (6 hours' time) × 12 per year			10-week session (15 hours' time) × 4 per year				
Group MNT hours (3)		72			60				
Estimated additional client care hours (4)	50	Estimated indirect hours (5)	575	Vacation/ relief coverage hours (6)	100	Total hours (7)	13,285	FTEs (8)	6.4

Abbreviations: ADA, American Dietetic Association; CKD, chronic kidney disease; DM, diabetes mellitus; FTEs, full-time equivalents; GDM, gestational diabetes mellitus; GFP, MNT Guide for Practice; HPL, hyperlipidemia; MNT, medical nutrition therapy; WM, weight management.

*MNT Guides for Practice are being developed. When published, check MNT Guide for Practice CD-ROMs for exact number of MNT hours.

Instructions:

1. Estimate the number of clients who will receive 1:1 MNT in the coming year, using past performance data and projected program goals.
2. Multiply the number of 1:1 clients by MNT hours from ADA MNT Guides for Practice and MNT Protocols. For diagnoses without protocols, multiply the number of 1:1 clients by estimated average MNT per client.
3. Estimate the number of MNT group sessions and hours of group MNT time.
4. Estimate the number of hours of additional client care—eg, additional MNT follow-up and prevention and wellness counseling (hours/month × 12).
5. Estimate the total indirect hours—eg, documentation, dietary analysis, meetings, program planning, marketing, and community presentations (hours/month × 12).
6. Estimate needed hours for relief coverage, if provided. Include vacation and professional and medical leaves.
7. Calculate total hours from all estimates, including 1:1 and group MNT hours.
8. Calculate FTEs required by dividing total hours by 2,080 hours (1 FTE).

Note: The template for this form is found in Appendix C.12.

Implementing a Staffing Plan: Worksheets

APPENDIX E.1   TEAM ACTIVITY: EVALUATING THE IMPACT OF CHANGES

Proposed Change:

List problems or unmet needs that exist as a result of the current situation:

1. _____

2. _____

3. _____

What problems does the current situation create for the work group I represent?

_____

_____

_____

_____

List three benefits or positive aspects of implementing the proposed program or staffing plan for the unit as a whole:

1. _____

2. _____

3. _____

How will these changes benefit the work group that I represent?

_____

_____

_____

_____

_____

_____

Note: For a completed example of this form, see Box 4.1.

APPENDIX E.2   IMPLEMENTATION PLAN

Performance Area	Strategies	Due Date	Responsibility	Progress
Internal Processes				
	Completion Date			
Finances				
	Completion Date			
Customers				
	Completion Date			

APPENDIX E.2   (*continued*)

Performance Area	Strategies	Due Date	Responsibility	Progress
Innovation and Learning				
	Completion Date			

Instructions:

1. Transfer "priorities for performance areas" to first column, from Balanced Scorecard Approach to Strategic Planning form (Appendix B.3).
2. Transfer strategies to achieve each performance area from Appendix B.3.
3. In collaboration with staff members and others who will implement the strategies, determine due dates and person(s) responsible for each strategy.
4. Use Progress column to record progress made toward implementing strategies listed.
5. List dates for completion of each set of performance area strategies.

Note: For a completed example of this form, see Figure 4.1.

APPENDIX E.3   OVERCOMING BARRIERS

Large-Group Activity: List the barriers that will need to be addressed when implementing the proposed changes.

Actual Barriers

1.

2.

3.

4.

5.

Potential Barriers

1.

2.

3.

4.

5.

Small-Group Activity: Divide into groups of two or three people. Assign one actual barrier to each small group.

Barrier_____

List ways to resolve the barrier. Specify actions to be taken and persons responsible for taking actions.

1.

2.

3.

4.

5.

6.

7.

Note: For completed examples of this form, see Boxes 4.2 and 4.3.

Measuring and Evaluating Staffing Effectiveness: Worksheets and Tools

APPENDIX F.1   ANNUAL PERFORMANCE TRACKING FORM

Work Area _____

	January	February	March	April	May	June	July	August	September	October	November	December	Year Totals
Direct care activity totals													
Actual UOS (1)													
Planned UOS (2)													
% variance (3)													
Facility data													
Total productivity factors (%) (4)													
Hours paid (5)													
Hours worked (6)													
Adjusted patient days (7)													
Outpatient data													
Actual charges (8)													
Planned charges (9)													
% variance (10)													
Outpatient UOS (11)													
Planned UOS (12)													
% variance (13)													

Abbreviation: UOS, units of service.

Instructions:

Direct Care Activity:

1. List actual UOS data from Direct Care Activity Summary form (Appendix F.8)—No. 9 on that form.
2. List planned UOS data from budget projections.
3. Calculate percentage variance: $100 - [(\text{Actual UOS/Planned UOS}) \times 100]$. List data.

Facility Data:

4. List total productivity factor (%) data from Direct Care Activity Summary form (Appendix F.8)—No. 8 on that form.
5. List monthly totals for hours paid from facility financial reports
6. List monthly totals for hours worked from facility financial reports.
7. List monthly totals for adjusted patient days from facility financial reports.

Outpatient Data:

8. List actual outpatient charges from Outpatient Direct Care Annual Summary Report (Appendix F.10).
9. List planned outpatient charges from budget projections.
10. Calculate percentage variance: $100 - [(\text{Actual charges/Planned charges}) \times 100]$. List data.
11. List outpatient UOS from Outpatient Direct Care Annual Summary Report (Appendix F.10).
12. List planned UOS from budget projections.
13. Calculate percentage variance: $100 - [(\text{Actual UOS/Planned UOS}) \times 100]$. List data.

Year Totals:

14. Determine year totals by adding each line across.

APPENDIX F.2   SUMMARY PERFORMANCE REPORT

Performance Indicators	Current Year	Trend	Benchmark	Comments
Internal processes				
Finances				
Customers				
Innovation and learning				

Instructions:

Use this report with the Balanced Scorecard Approach to Strategic Planning form (Appendix B.3) to describe annual department performance. List performance indicators from Appendix B.3, current year performance, trends (up, down, no change), and benchmark targets. Note factors that affected results under Comments.

APPENDIX F.3   STAFFING PLAN EVALUATION FORM

Use this form to evaluate actual staffing vs planned staffing, as described in Chapter 5.

Week of _____

Dates								Averages
Registered dietitian FTEs planned								
Registered dietitian FTEs worked								
% compliance								1
Dietetic technician FTEs planned								
Dietetic technician FTEs worked								
% compliance								2
Total clinical staff FTEs planned								
Total clinical staff FTEs worked								
% compliance								3

Instructions:

1. For a 1-week period, list the number of dietitian, dietetic technician, and total clinical staff FTEs shown on the staff schedule and the number of FTEs of each position actually worked, obtained from payroll reports.
2. Calculate percentage compliance by dividing the number of planned or scheduled FTEs by the number of worked FTEs and multiplying result by 100.
3. Add the numbers of planned/scheduled and worked FTEs for dietitians, dietetic technicians, and clinical staff; divide result by 7; and list average number of FTEs scheduled and worked in final column.
4. Add the compliance percentages for each day and divide by 7.
5. Transfer compliance averages (Boxes 1–3) for each week audited to the Staffing Plan Evaluation: Summary of Compliance form (Appendix F.4) and the compliance averages for dietitians and dietetic technicicans (Boxes 1 and 2) to the Human Resources Indicator Matrix (Appendix F.14).

APPENDIX F.4   STAFFING PLAN EVALUATION: SUMMARY OF COMPLIANCE

Use this form to evaluate actual staffing vs planned staffing, as described in Chapter 5.

Weeks										Averages
% compliance: registered dietitians										
% compliance: dietetic technicians										
% compliance: total clinical nutrition staff										

Instructions:

1. List average compliance percentages for dietitians, dietetic technicians, and total clinical nutrition staff for each week audited.

2. Add average compliance percentages, divide by the number of weeks audited, and list overall averages in final column.

APPENDIX F.5 DIRECT CARE ACTIVITY TRACKING FORM

Dietitians and dietetic technicians use this form to record the number of activities completed each week, as described in Chapter 5.

RD _____

Dates	Nutrition Screening	Nutrition Assessment: MR	Nutrition Assessment: HR	Reassessment: MR	Reassessment: HR	Calorie Counts HR	MR	Basic Education HR	MR	Complex Education HR	MR
Monday											
Tuesday											
Wednesday											
Thursday											
Friday											
Saturday											
Sunday											
Totals											

Abbreviations: HR, high risk; MR, moderate risk.

Instructions:

1. List the number of each activity by date. List the total number for each activity completed for the week in the last row. Transfer the totals to the Direct Care Activity Individual Summary form (Appendix F.7).
2. The Clinical Effectiveness Tracking form (Appendix F.18) can be filled out at the same time that this form is completed.

APPENDIX F.6 DIRECT CARE ACTIVITY TRACKING FORM (WITH NUTRITION DIAGNOSES)

Dietitians and dietetic technicians use this form to record the number of activities completed each week, as described in Chapter 5.

RD _____

Dates	Nutrition Screening	Nutrition Assessment: MR	Nutrition Assessment: HR	Nutrition Diagnosis: Weight Loss*	Nutrition Diagnosis: Inadequate Intake*	Reassessment: MR	Reassessment: HR	Calorie Counts HR	Calorie Counts MR	Basic Education HR	Basic Education MR	Complex Education HR	Complex Education MR
Monday													
Tuesday													
Wednesday													
Thursday													
Friday													
Saturday													
Sunday													
Totals													

Abbreviations: HR, high risk; MR, moderate risk.

*List the number of patients who received high-risk nutrition assessment and who had a nutrition diagnosis of weight loss and/or inadequate intake. List patients with both nutrition diagnoses in both columns. These numbers will provide an overall estimate of the relative proportions of high-risk patients with these two nutrition diagnoses.

Instructions:

1. List the number of each activity performed by date. List the total number of each activity completed for the week in the last row.
2. Transfer the totals to the "Direct Care Activity Individual Summary" form (Appendix F.7).

APPENDIX F.7 DIRECT CARE ACTIVITY INDIVIDUAL SUMMARY FORM

Dietitians and dietetic technicians use this form to summarize the number of activities completed each month and the time spent on activities, as described in Chapter 5.

Name _____

Month _____

Dates	Nutrition Screening	Nutrition Assessment: MR	Nutrition Assessment: High Risk (HRA)	Reassessment MR	Reassessment HR	Calorie Counts		Basic Education		Complex Education	
						HR	MR	HR	MR	HR	MR
Activity totals (1)											
× Activity factors (2)											
= Total time per activity (hours) (3)											
HRAs w/weight loss diagnosis (4)	HRAs w/inadequate intake diagnosis (5)		Total direct care time (6)		Total paid time (7)			Productivity factor (%) (8)			
No.: _____ %	No.: _____ %										

Abbreviations: HR, high risk; HRA, high-risk assessment; MR, moderate risk.

Instructions (for Appendix F.7, p. 221):

Use weekly totals from the Direct Care Activity Tracking forms (Appendixes F.5 or F.6) to do the following:

1. List monthly totals for activities.
2. Insert activity factors.
3. Multiply each activity total by its activity factor.
4. List number of HRAs with nutrition diagnosis of weight loss, as well as percentage of total HRAs completed.
5. List number of HRAs with nutrition diagnosis of inadequate intake, as well as percentage of total HRAs completed.
6. Add time totals for each activity from "Total time per activity" row.
7. Obtain total paid time from payroll report or calculate.
8. Calculate productivity factor (%): (Total direct care time ÷ Total paid time) × 100.

APPENDIX F.8 DIRECT CARE ACTIVITY SUMMARY FORM

Month _____

Dates	Nutrition Screening	Nutrition Assessment: MR	Nutrition Assessment: High Risk (HRA)	Reassessment MR	Reassessment HR	Calorie Counts HR	Calorie Counts MR	Basic Education HR	Basic Education MR	Complex Education HR	Complex Education MR
Activity totals (1)											
× Activity factors (2)											
= Total time per activity (hours) (3)			A	B	C			D		E	

HRAs w/weight loss diagnosis (4)	HRAs w/inadequate intake diagnosis (5)	Total direct care time (6)	Total paid time (7)	Productivity factor (%) (8)	Total UOS (9)	High-Risk DC time (10)	High-Risk UOS (11)
No.: ____ %	No.: ____ %						

Abbreviations: DC, direct care; HR, high risk; HRA, high-risk assessment; MR, moderate risk; UOS, units of service.

Instructions (for Appendix F.8, p. 223):

Use weekly totals from the Direct Care Activity Individual Summary forms (Appendix F.7) to do the following:

1. List monthly totals for activities.
2. Insert activity factors.
3. Multiply each activity total by its activity factor.
4. List number of HRAs with nutrition diagnosis of weight loss, as well as percentage of total HRAs completed.
5. List number of HRAs with nutrition diagnosis of inadequate intake, as well as percentage of total HRAs completed.
6. Add time totals for each activity from "Total time per activity" row.
7. Obtain total paid time from payroll report or calculate.
8. Calculate productivity factor: (Total direct care time ÷ Total paid time) × 100.
9. Calculate total UOS: Total direct care time × 4. (1 UOS = 15 minutes; 4 UOS per hour.)
10. Calculate high-risk DC time: A + B + C + D + E.
11. Calculate high-risk UOS: High-risk DC time × 4.

APPENDIX F.9 OUTPATIENT DIRECT CARE TRACKING FORM

RD _____

1 UOS = 15 minutes

Diagnosis or Clinic	January	February	March	April	May	June	July	August	September	October	November	December	Year Totals
Initial													
Follow-up													
Initial													
Follow-up													
Initial													
Follow-up													
Other—initial													
Other—follow-up													
Total UOS									Total annual UOS				
Charges ($)											Total annual charges		

Abbreviation: UOS, units of service.

Instructions:

1. List number of UOS by clinic site or diagnosis for a breakdown of the type of work performed/care provided.
2. Transfer monthly staff totals to Outpatient Direct Care Annual Summary Report (Appendix F.10).

APPENDIX F.10 OUTPATIENT DIRECT CARE ANNUAL SUMMARY REPORT

RD Names	January UOS	January $	February UOS	February $	March UOS	March $	April UOS	April $	May UOS	May $	June UOS	June $	July UOS	July $	August UOS	August $	September UOS	September $	October UOS	October $	November UOS	November $	December UOS	December $
	January		February		March		April		May		June		July		August		September		October		November		December	
Total monthly UOS															Total annual UOS									
Total monthly charges ($)																	Total annual charges							

Abbreviation: UOS, units of service.

Instructions:

List UOS and charges for each registered dietitian (RD) by month (monthly totals are tracked with Outpatient Direct Care Tracking Form found in Appendix F.9).

APPENDIX F.11   NUTRITION SCREENING AUDIT

Use this form with forms in Appendixes F.12 and F.13 to monitor completion of nutrition care processes, as described in Chapter 5.

MR No.	Admission Date	Screening Completed		Date of Screening	Time Standard Met		Consultation Sent			Rescreening Completed			Time Standard Met		Comments
		Yes	No		Yes	No	Yes	No	N/A	Yes	No	N/A	Yes	No	
Total no. of charts audited	Totals														
	Compliance %														

Instructions:

List data in the columns indicated. Calculate the total number of assessments completed, totals met and not met for each audit area, and compliance percentages for each audit area.

APPENDIX F.12   NUTRITION ASSESSMENT AUDIT

Use this form with Appendixes F.11 and F.13 to monitor completion of nutrition care processes, as described in Chapter 5.

Audit Date _____ Unit _____

RD _____

MR No.	Admission or Consultation Date	Date of Nutrition Assessment	Nutritional Risk Level		Nutrition Assessment Time Standard Met		Nutrition Diagnosis Documented		Specific and Timed Goals in Plan		Comments
			High	Moderate	Yes	No	Yes	No	Yes	No	
Total assessments completed		Totals									
		Compliance %									

Instructions:

List data in the columns indicated. Calculate the total number of assessments completed, totals met and not met for each audit area, and compliance percentages for each audit area.

APPENDIX F.13   NUTRITION REASSESSMENT AUDIT

Use this form with Appendixes F.11 and F.12 to monitor completion of nutrition care processes, as described in Chapter 5.

Audit Date _____   Unit _____

RD _____

MR No.	Date of Prior Assessment	Date of Nutrition Reassessment	Nutritional Risk Level		Nutrition Reassessment Time Standard Met		Evaluation of Goal Progress		Specific and Timed Goals in Plan		Comments
			High	Moderate	Yes	No	Yes	No	Yes	No	
Total reassessments completed	Totals										
	Compliance %										

Instructions:

List data in the columns indicated. Calculate the total number of reassessments completed, totals met and not met for each audit area, and compliance percentages for each audit area.

APPENDIX F.14   HUMAN RESOURCES INDICATOR MATRIX

Work Area _____

	January	February	March	April	May	June	July	August	September	October	November	December	Annual Average
% compliance w/staffing plan: RDs (1)													
% compliance w/staffing plan: total clinical nutrition staff (2)													
Worked RD hours per APD (3)													
Worked technician hours per APD (4)													
Paid RD hours per APD (5)													
Paid technician hours per APD (6)													
Total staff worked hours per APD (7)													
Total paid hours per APD (8)													
Staff vacancy rate (9)													

Abbreviations: APD, adjusted patient days; FTE, full-time equivalent; RD, registered dietitian.

Instructions

1. Transfer data on percentage of compliance with staffing plan by RDs from Staffing Plan Evaluation form (Appendix F.3).
2. Transfer data on percentage of compliance with staffing plan by total clinical nutrition staff from Staffing Plan Evaluation form (Appendix F.3).
3. Obtain RD worked hours from the facility's financial reports. Calculate: RD worked hours divided by APD from the Annual Performance Tracking form (Appendix F.1).
4. Obtain technician worked hours from the facility's financial reports. Calculate: technician worked hours divided by APD from the Annual Performance Tracking form (Appendix F.1).
5. Obtain RD paid hours from the facility's financial reports. Calculate: RD paid hours divided by APD from data on the Annual Performance Tracking form (Appendix F.1).
6. Obtain technician paid hours from the facility's financial reports. Calculate: technician paid hours divided by APD from data on the Annual Performance Tracking form (Appendix F.1).
7. Obtain total worked hours from the Annual Performance Tracking form (Appendix F.1) or the facility's financial reports.
8. Obtain total paid hours from the Annual Performance Tracking form (Appendix F.1) or the facility's financial reports.
9. Calculate monthly staff vacancy rate: $100 - [(\text{Actual FTEs} \div \text{Budgeted FTE}) \times 100]$.

APPENDIX F.15   SERVICE INDICATOR MATRIX

Work Area _____

	January	February	March	April	May	June	July	August	September	October	November	December	Annual Average
Total UOS or direct care activities per APD (12)													
High-risk UOS or direct care activities per APD (13)													
Total direct care time per APD (14)													
Total high-risk patient direct care time per APD (15)													
% compliance w/high-risk assessment time standard (16)													
% compliance w/high-risk reassessment time standard (17)													

Abbreviations: APD, adjusted patient days; UOS, units of service.

Instructions:

12. Obtain total UOS from the Direct Care Activity Summary form (Appendix F.8)—No. 9 on that form. Obtain APD from the Annual Performance Tracking form (Appendix F.1) or the facility's financial reports.

13. Obtain high-risk UOS from the Direct Care Activity Summary form (Appendix F.9)—No. 11 on that form. Obtain APD from the Annual Performance Tracking form (Appendix F.1) or the facility's financial reports.

14. Obtain total direct care times from the Direct Care Activity Summary form (Appendix F.8)—No. 6 on that form. Obtain APD from the "Annual Performance Tracking" form (Appendix F.1) or the facility's financial reports.

15. Obtain high-risk direct care times from the Direct Care Activity Summary form (Appendix F.8)— No. 10 on that form. Obtain APD from the "Annual Performance Tracking" form (Appendix F.1) or the facility's financial reports.

16. Calculate compliance percentage using data from monthly chart audits from Nutrition Assessment Audit form (Appendix F.12): (No. of charts with assessments meeting established time standards ÷ Total no. of audited charts with assessments) × 100.

17. Calculate compliance percentage using data from monthly chart audits from Nutrition Reassessment Audit form (Appendix F.13): (No. of charts with reassessments meeting established time standards ÷ Total no. of audited charts with reassessments) × 100.

APPENDIX F.16 CLINICAL INDICATOR MATRIX

Work Area _____

	January	February	March	April	May	June	July	August	September	October	November	December	Annual Average
% improvement in weight-loss nutrition diagnosis (I)													
% improvement in inadequate-intake nutrition diagnosis (J)													
% nutrition care plan weight goal met (K) (high-risk patients with weight-loss diagnosis)													
% nutrition care plan intake goal met (L) (high-risk patients with inadequate intake diagnosis)													
% energy requirements met (M) (high-risk patients with inadequate intake diagnosis)													
% protein requirements met (N) (high-risk patients with inadequate intake diagnosis)													

Instructions:

Transfer data from monthly Clinical Effectiveness Tracking Form—Department/Unit Summary forms (Appendix F.20).

APPENDIX F.17 STAFFING EFFECTIVENESS INDICATOR MATRIX: CORE MEASURES

Work Area _____

	January	February	March	April	May	June	July	August	September	October	November	December	Annual Average
Human Resources													
% RD days compliance w/ staffing plan (1)													
Paid RD hours per APD (5)													
Service													
High-risk UOS or direct care activities per APD (13)													
Total high-risk patient direct care time per APD (15)													
Clinical													
% improvement in weight-loss nutrition diagnosis (I)													
% improvement in inadequate - intake nutrition diagnosis (J)													

Abbreviations: APD, adjusted patient days; RD, registered dietitian; UOS, units of service.

Instructions (for Appendix F.17, p. 235):

The core measures are focused on the nutrition care provided to high-risk patients. Therefore, use RD staffing plan compliance, high-risk direct care time, and UOS of high-risk direct care activities completed, so that comparison of the three types of indicator data is specific to the same group of patients (ie, patients at high nutrition risk who receive nutrition care from RDs). Obtain 1 and 5 from the Human Resources Indicator Matrix (Appendix F.14), 13 and 15 from the Service Indicator Matrix (Appendix F.15), and I and J from the Clinical Indicator Matrix (Appendix F.16).

APPENDIX F.18   CLINICAL EFFECTIVENESS TRACKING FORM

RD _____

Dates	Nutrition Reassessments: High Risk (1)	Nutrition Diagnosis: Weight Loss (2)	Improvement: Nutrition Diagnosis of Weight Loss (3)	Weight Goal in Nutrition Care Plan Met (4)	Nutrition Diagnosis: Inadequate Intake (5)	Improvement: Nutrition Diagnosis of Inadequate Intake (6)	Intake Goal in Nutrition Care Plan Met (7)	Energy Requirement Met (8)	Protein Requirement Met (9)
Monday									
Tuesday									
Wednesday									
Thursday									
Friday									
Saturday									
Sunday									
Totals									

Instructions (for Appendix F.18, p. 237):

1. List the total number of patients receiving high-risk nutrition reassessments.
2. List the number of patients receiving high-risk nutrition reassessments who had a nutrition diagnosis of weight loss.
3. List the number of patients with a nutrition diagnosis of weight loss who had improvements in the signs and symptoms of this diagnosis.
4. List the number of patients with a nutrition diagnosis of weight loss who met the weight goal that was established in the most recently documented nutrition care plan.
5. List the number of patients receiving high-risk nutrition reassessments who had a nutrition diagnosis of inadequate intake.
6. List the number of patients with a nutrition diagnosis of inadequate intake who had improvements in the signs and symptoms of this diagnosis.
7. List the number of patients with a nutrition diagnosis of inadequate intake who met the intake goal that was established in the most recently documented nutrition care plan.
8. List the number of patients with a nutrition diagnosis of inadequate intake who met their estimated energy requirement at the time of the reassessment.
9. List the number of patients with a nutrition diagnosis of inadequate intake who met their estimated protein requirement at the time of the reassessment.

This form allows staff to use data collected during nutrition reassessment of high-risk patients to evaluate the impact of nutrition intervention on the following:

- *Improvements in the signs and symptoms of two nutrition diagnoses,* weight loss and inadequate intake, identified during an initial nutrition assessment or a previous reassessment.
- *Ability to meet the goals for weight and intake* that were established in a nutrition care plan from a prior nutrition assessment or reassessment.
- *Ability to meet calculated energy and protein requirements* as determined on the day of the reassessment [(Actual intake ÷ Estimated requirement) × 100]. Definition of "meets requirements" is facility specific but may be set at 85% of requirements or higher.

The comparison is made between the total number of patients receiving reassessment who had a prior diagnosis of either weight loss or inadequate intake and the number of patients with improvements, as listed above. To use this system, RDs must use the Nutrition Care Process (passed by the American Dietetic Association House of Delegates in May 2003) and, at a minimum, identify these two nutrition diagnoses or problems, as described in step 2 in the Nutrition Care Process.

Complete this form at the same time as the Direct Care Activity Tracking (with nutrition diagnoses) form (Appendix F.6).

APPENDIX F.19   CLINICAL EFFECTIVENESS TRACKING FORM—INDIVIDUAL SUMMARY

Month _____

RD _____

Dates: List Totals for Each Week	Nutrition Reassessments: High Risk (1)	Nutrition Diagnosis: Weight Loss (2)	Improvement: Nutrition Diagnosis of Weight Loss (3)	Weight Goal in Nutrition Care Plan Met (4)	Nutrition Diagnosis: Inadequate Intake (5)	Improvement: Nutrition Diagnosis of Inadequate Intake (6)	Intake Goal in Nutrition Care Plan Met (7)	Energy Requirement Met (8)	Protein Requirement Met (9)
Monthly Totals									

Instructions:

Transfer the weekly totals for each column from the "Clinical Effectiveness Tracking" forms (Appendix F.18). In a typical month, there will be four to five sets of weekly totals.

APPENDIX F.20   CLINICAL EFFECTIVENESS TRACKING FORM—INDIVIDUAL SUMMARY

Month _____   RD _____

Dates: List Totals for Each Registered Dietitian (RD)	Nutrition Reassessments: High Risk (1)	Nutrition Diagnosis: Weight Loss (2)	Improvement: Nutrition Diagnosis of Weight Loss (3)	Weight Goal in Nutrition Care Plan Met (4)	Nutrition Diagnosis: Inadequate Intake (5)	Improvement: Nutrition Diagnosis of Inadequate Intake (6)	Intake Goal in Nutrition Care Plan Met (7)	Energy Requirement Met (8)	Protein Requirement Met (9)
Monthly totals (all staff)	A	B		C	D	E	F	G	H
Clinical indicator rates	$B/A \times 100 = I$			$C/A \times 100 = K$	$K =$	$E/D \times 100 = J$	$J =$	$F/D \times 100 = L$	$H/D \times 100 = N$
	$I =$					$G/D \times 100 = M$	$M =$	$L =$	$N =$

Instructions:

Transfer the monthly RD totals from the Clinical Effectiveness Tracking Form—Individual Summary (Appendix F.19). Transfer the clinical indicator rates to the Clinical Indicator Matrix (Appendix F.16).

APPENDIX F.21   SELECTING PERFORMANCE INDICATORS

Indicators	Data Available	High Volume	Problem Prone	Clinical Impact	Total Points
Human Resources					
Percentage of days in compliance with staffing plan					
RD and/or DT paid hours per adjusted patient days					
RD and/or DT worked hours per adjusted patient days					
Clinical nutrition staff vacancy rate					
Service					
Units of service per adjusted patient days (all patients or high-risk patients only)					
Hours of direct care time per adjusted patient days (all patients or high-risk patients only)					
Percentage compliance with time standard for completion of high-risk nutrition assessments					
Percentage compliance with time standard for completion of high-risk nutrition monitoring and reassessment					
Clinical					
Percentage improvement between initial and follow-up assessments for nutrition diagnoses of weight loss (high-risk patients)					
Percentage improvement between initial and follow-up assessments for nutrition diagnoses of inadequate intake (high-risk patients)					
Percentage achievement of nutrient requirements between initial assessment and reassessment (high-risk patients)					
Percentage achievement of nutrition care plan goals between initial assessment and reassessment (high-risk patients)					

Scoring system: High, 3 points; medium, 2 points; low, 1 point.

Instructions:

Use this form to select core measures for evaluating staffing effectiveness.

1. In the columns for each indicator, list a numeric score based on an evaluation of facility-specific factors that affect the indicator. For example, data available = 3; high volume = 3; problem prone = 1; clinical impact = 3.
2. Add the points for each indicator across and record in column for total points.
3. Select the one or two core measures with the highest point totals in each of the three sections (Human Resources, Service, and Clinical) to track and monitor on an ongoing basis. Evaluation of all three types of indicators is part of a "Balanced Scorecard Approach" to determining staffing effectiveness.

APPENDIX F.22 OUTCOMES PROJECT CHECKLIST

When planning an outcomes project, include the following components:

1. **Practice question**—a question not answered by existing evidence. Use the PICO format (P = patient group; I = intervention; C = control or comparison group; O = outcome or outcomes).
2. **Review of literature**
3. **Study design**
   - Comparison to be made
     - Intervention to be tested
     - Comparison group care
   - Sample
     - Description
     - Inclusion and exclusion criteria
     - Sample size
   - Data to be collected
     - Patient characteristics
     - Details of the care process/intervention
   - Outcome indicators and tools/methods to measure outcomes
     - Covariates and confounders—factors that can affect outcomes
   - Frequency of data collection

4. **Study methods**
   - Enrollment
     - Recruitment
     - Screening for eligibility—also track patients who are screened but not enrolled
     - Consent process
     - Assignment to intervention and comparison groups
   - Standard methods
     - Procedures—consider creating a study manual
       - Care process
       - Accountability for data collection
       - Timing of data collection during care process—the logistics
     - Forms and tools—include copies in the manual
     - Definitions of terms
     - Potential for bias of results—removal of sources of bias
     - Sites
       - One location versus multiple sites
       - Commitment—initial approval and ongoing commitment
       - Institutional review board approval
       - Training and retraining of staff
       - Communication
     - Plans for pilot
     - Data accuracy
     - Plans to check data collection during study

5. Data analysis and reporting
- Database or spreadsheet
- Coding and data entry
- Statistical analysis
  - ➤ Summary data
  - ➤ Testing of hypothesis of the effect of intervention
  - ➤ Adjustment for covariates
- Plans for presentation and publication
- Use of data in practice setting to improve patient care and market the use of medical nutrition therapy/registered dietitians

6. Timeline
- Due dates for completing each component of the project
- Regular reassessment of progress

Source: Data are from American Dietetic Association Scientific Affairs and Research. *ADA Evidence Analysis Guide.* 2nd ed. Chicago, Ill: American Dietetic Association; 2003.

Index